SPEECH AFTER STROKE

SPEECH AFTER STROKE

A MANUAL FOR THE
SPEECH PATHOLOGIST
AND THE FAMILY MEMBER
Second Edition

By

STEPHANIE STRYKER, M.A.

Certified Speech Pathologist
Consultant, Mt. Sinai Medical Center, Miami Heart Institute
St. Francis, Mercy, North Miami General, Parkway General and
Osteopathic General Hospitals, Miami, Florida

With a Foreword by
Jon Eisenson, Ph.D.

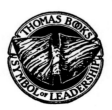

CHARLES C THOMAS · PUBLISHER
Springfield · Illinois · U.S.A.

Published and Distributed Throughout the World by

CHARLES C THOMAS · PUBLISHER

Bannerstone House

301–327 East Lawrence Avenue, Springfield, Illinois, U.S.A.

© 1975, 1981 *by* STEPHANIE STRYKER

ISBN 0-398-04122-9

Library of Congress Catalog Card Number: 80-17949

First Edition, 1975
Second Edition, 1981

Library of Congress Cataloging in Publication Data

Stryker, Stephanie.
  Speech after stroke.

  Bibliography: p.
  Includes index.
  1. Stroke patients — Rehabilitation. 2. Speech
therapy. I. Title. [DNLM: 1. Aphasia — Therapy.
2. Cerebrovascular disorders. 3. Speech disorders
— Rehabilitation. WL355 S928s]
RC388.5.S86 1980   616.8'1   80-17949
ISBN 0-398-04122-9

Printed in the United States of America

C-1

ACKNOWLEDGMENTS

Dale Stryker, M.S., Illustrator
The author takes pride in acknowledging her talented sister, Dale, who designed all of the illustrations. Her creativeness and artistic ability is evidenced by her graphically clear depictions which compliment the text. She is currently employed as an art teacher in the Dade County Public Schools. Miami, Florida. Many thanks for an excellent job!

Susan R. Cohen, B.A., Editorial Consultant
The author thanks her dear friend and editorial consultant, Sue, for her excellent suggestions and expertise in preparation of the manuscript regarding general organization and structure, and logical order of presentation of contents. She spent many hours with me, collating the material, indexing, and putting the manuscript into final form. I am deply grateful for her help.

Eleanor Stryker Toch, Manuscript Typist
The author wishes to express heartfelt thanks to her mother, Eleanor, who spent many long hours typing the entire manuscript. In addition, she made many innovative suggestions regarding revisions and additions to the wording of the text. Her encouragement and support throughout this project has been invaluable.

FOREWORD

Language clinicians working with aphasic patients are usually very busy people, ever on the lookout for materials that can be directly used or modified for use with their clients. Ms. Stryker's handbook *Speech After Stroke* is a useful collection of materials that can reduce the burden of search for the clinician.

I am particularly impressed with the potentials of the material for individual adaptation, especially in the early stages of therapy. The basic principle for the selection of materials is that of practicability. The materials are there because they have been found to produce results.

There is much that provides a basis for using the contents as points of departure and as prototypes for a clinician using individual imagination and creative ability to produce "exercises" specific to the needs of a particular patient. Nothing in this manual interferes with a clinician's creativity in the development of materials. In brief, the material is not prescriptive but representative of what a practicing speech pathologist with considerable experience with aphasic patients has found useful.

Jon Eisenson, Ph.D.

CONTENTS

PREFACE

"WHAT CAN I DO TO HELP MY HUSBAND OR WIFE SPEAK AGAIN?"

THIS QUESTION, which is heard repeatedly by the speech pathologist, prompted the writing of this book and dictates its contents. The purpose of this manual is to provide the speech pathologist and the untrained family members with structured practice material which can be used in helping the aphasic patient recover language and speech skills impaired due to a brain injury, commonly referred to as a "stroke." A brain injury may be caused by a vascular accident, trauma to the head, or a space-occupying lesion (tumor), etc. The loss of language skills due to any of these causes is termed "aphasia." Aphasia impairs communication ability, i.e. it affects a person's ability to comprehend, read, tell time, calculate, write, and speak. The degree to which these functions are impaired ranges from mild to severe and varies from patient to patient. Speech pathology treatment has proven to be helpful in the rehabilitation of these aphasic language disturbances.

Unfortunately, there is a paucity of material available commercially which is structured in a way that is simple enough yet suitable for the brain-injured adult without being childish. Presenting the adult aphasic patient with infantile picture cards and elementary word-phase drills can only result in devastating humiliation. The choice of words and pictures used in this manual was determined by their appropriateness for adults. The materials are relevant to the adult patient's everyday needs and activities. The exercises have been printed in bold-face, lower-case type for ease of reading to accommodate those with reduced visual acuity. In order to stimulate maximum vocabulary recall, the illustrations were organized into categories, e.g. "Grooming," "Clothing," "Food," "Drinks," "Furniture," etc. It is felt that grouping illustrated words into categories would enhance language recall by the process of association of words within the same class.

This book is divided into five main sections. Within each section, the items have been arranged so as to progress from the simple to the more complex material. Each section is subdivided as follows:

Section #1 COMPREHENSION OF THE SPOKEN WORD
    A) Following commands
    B) Pointing to objects, body parts, and pictures
    C) Use of gestures and nodding the head "yes" and "no"
    D) Use of a "communication board"
Section #2 IMITATIVE ABILITY AND ARTICULATION DRILLS
    A) Strengthening the oral musculature — tongue and lip exercises
    B) Repetition practice — Lists of words and sentences of increasing length
    C) Articulation drills for individual consonant sounds
Section #3 VOCABULARY RECALL, GRAMMAR AND SYNTAX
    A) Fill-in tasks and sentence completion
    B) Illustrated useful objects in categories
    C) Grammar usage and proper word order drills
    D) Advanced fill-in sentences in paragraphs
Section #4 READING DEVELOPMENT SKILLS
    A) Comprehension of written material
    B) Oral reading of words and useful phrases, phonic drills — words that look similar
    C) Money concepts
    D) Time-telling practice with illustrated clocks
    E) Advanced oral reading selections
Section #5 WRITING DEVELOPMENT SKILLS
    A) Copying
    B) Writing to dictation
    C) Writing from memory
    D) Advanced writing

There is no set recommended time limit to be spent on each of these sections. Rather, when the patient is successful on an individual exercise, it is suggested that he progress to the next exercise, thus, the orientation for these exercises is the patient's needs, not a time framework. The importance of follow-up practice by the patient with his family cannot be over-emphasized.

It is best to start aphasia rehabilitation as soon as possible after the brain injury. Your physician will advise you when he feels the patient is ready to begin. If a patient is unwilling to cooperate with the speech pathologist, he should not be forced to continue. Motivation and willingness on the part of the patient plays an important role in the patient's success.

The words speech pathologist, clinician, and family member are used interchangeably throughout this manual for purposes of simplicity. It should be obvious however, that the terms speech pathologist and clinician refer to a professional person with specific clinical training. It is highly recommended that a speech pathologist/language clinician treat the aphasic patient. However, an untrained family member, nurse, or friend can act as an assistant to reinforce learning, using these materials as a guide.

The author encourages the clinician to improvise and expand these materials so as to adapt them to the specific needs of the individual patients.

INTRODUCTION

TYPES OF SPEECH AND LANGUAGE DISORDERS

There are three major types of speech and language disorders resulting from brain damage. They are—

1. *Aphasia*—a breakdown in language skills resulting in impaired comprehension of the spoken and written word (receptive language) as well as impaired speech, gestures, and written language (expressive language). There is a reduction of available vocabulary and word recall, demonstrated by the patient's difficulty naming items and expressing ideas, and impaired grammar usage and syntax (word order).
2. *Dysarthria*—impaired speech pronunciation due to oral musculature weakness. Speech is characterized by slurred imprecise articulation. Rate is altered; tongue movements are usually labored. Voice quality may be abnormal, i.e. hypernasal; volume may be weak; drooling and swallowing and breathing difficulties may be present. Dysarthria may either accompany aphasia or occur alone.
3. *Verbal Apraxia*—Impaired repetition and imitative ability; lack of voluntary control and proper sequencing of articulators (tongue, lips, jaws, and vocal folds). Speech is characterized by sound reversals, additions, and word approximations due to sensorimotor impairment. The ability to imitate oral movements on command and to repeat words and phases is impaired although there is no accompanying weakness of the oral musculature. Verbal apraxia often accompanies aphasia.

EVALUATING THE EXTENT OF THE DISORDER

In order to determine the extent and type of disorder and in order to assess the potential for relearning, the patient should be evaluated by a certified speech pathologist. The physician in charge of the case will most likely be able to recommend a local certified speech pathologist. If not, a list of such individuals is available by writing to the American Speech-Language-Hearing Association, 10801 Rockville Pike, Rockville, MD 20852.

The speech evaluation serves several purposes: First, it reveals the patient's present speech capabilities; second, based on the patient's test performance, an individualized treatment program can then be planned; third, even if the speech pathologist is unable to administer the follow-up care, he will discuss the results of the evaluation so as to guide the family members in knowing at what level to begin speech rehabilitation and how to proceed using this manual.

ADMINISTERING APHASIA THERAPY

The recommended procedures for administering speech pathology treatment to the aphasic patient are as follows:

1. *Tell the patient why he is having this speech difficulty.* Explain to him in simple terms that he has suffered a brain injury and that this is the cause of his speech and language difficulty. Many patients have actually said that they think they are "going crazy." This is of course not true and should be made clear to the patient to avoid further frustration.

2. *Encourage and reassure the patient that he is likely to improve.* Most stoke patients do improve; however, improvement usually takes many months or more.

3. *Be patient.* Avoid scolding or shouting at the patient while urging him to respond. One must realize that most patients are trying their best. They are not purposely withholding information, but rather are displaying reduced vocabulary. Many are depressed and need support rather than chiding. Not all family members can work well as an assistant. If a person's temperament is such that he is impatient, nervous, overanxious, or intolerant, this person should not work with the patient.

4. *Speak slowly to the aphasic patient.* Patients with brain damage often have input difficulties and consequently need more time to assimilate information. A patient with a comprehension deficit hears but doesn't fully understand what is being said to him. It is much the same as listening to a foreign language when in a foreign country. The patient hears the words, but he requires slow presentation of the material so that he can grasp the material better.

5. *Use simple concrete language.* Ask straightforward questions to avoid unnecessary confusion. For example, say "Do you want coffee?"—"yes or no?" (Wait for the patient's response.) "Do you want tea?"—rather than asking the more complex question, "Do you want coffee, tea, or would you prefer milk?"

6. *Make realistic goals and expectations.* Avoid demanding too

much of the patient. If a person cannot name things, demanding words and full sentences is not a realistic goal for beginning treatment.

7. *Give the patient ample time to respond.* If given enough time, many patients can elicit the correct response. It is much the same as when a person has the word on the tip of his tongue, so to speak; if given enough time, often he will be able to evoke the proper response.

8. *Begin practice sessions at a level where the patient can feel successful.* Graduate slowly upward to more difficult levels. Avoid haphazard drilling, in which the family member attempts not only to cover too much material but also does this without a logical sequence or presentation. A patient should not be subjected to a speech pathology session in which all of the material presented is too difficult for him. A frustrated patient easily becomes disinterested, fatigued and, depressed. On the other hand, a successful patient will be more cooperative and be more likely to progress.

9. *Watch for signs of fatigue and perseveration.* Perseveration means repetition of an act or word after it is no longer appropriate. Brain-injured patients often display perseveration and shortened attention span. These signs indicate a need for a change of activity. Usually stopping and resting for awhile or changing the subject is helpful.

10. *Keep treatment sessions short and at frequent intervals.* This, of course, depends on the individual's attention span, but most often a fifteen- to twenty-minute practice session two to three times a day is better than one hour-long session.

11. *Treat the patient as a adult, not a child.* Even though he may be unable to communicate effectively, and may at times display childlike behavior, e.g. uncontrolled or inappropriate crying or laughing caused by the brain injury, he should not be ridiculed or babied.

Oftentimes, well meaning friends who may have experienced similar circumstances with stroke patients may attempt to impose their own ideas on your family member. Although their intentions are good, one must remember that each patient is unique and treatment procedures may vary. Following the above recommended procedures will provide guidelines for treatment. The exercises should be adapted to suit the patient's particular interests and needs.

SPEECH AFTER STROKE

COMPREHENSION OF THE SPOKEN WORD

A)   Following commands

B)   Pointing to objects, body parts, and pictures

C)   Use of gestures—nodding "yes and no"

D)   Use of a communication board

COMPREHENSION OF THE SPOKEN WORD

T HE RECOVERY OF LANGUAGE depends mainly upon the patient's ability to understand and follow directions and upon the scope and severity of his illness. The relearning of expressive speech and language skills cannot occur unless the patient can comprehend the speech pathologist's instructions. Most patients who have aphasia usually demonstrate some impairment in auditory comprehension, that is, impairment in understanding the spoken word. This impairment may range from minimal to severe. During the initial evaluation an assessment is made of the patient's comprehension abilities in order to determine if he is an appropriate candidate for rehabilitation and at what level the treatment should begin.

Very often a patient may appear to understand conversational speech by nodding his head and smiling. However, when asked to follow specific simple commands, he may be unable to do so. Although it is difficult for the family to accept the fact that their loved one cannot comprehend as he did prior to the brain injury, it is in the best interests of the patient for one to be realistic about his deficit. It should be kept in mind, however, that improvement in comprehension often occurs spontaneously, and even though the improvement in some cases may be more gradual, for example, over a period of several months, most patients do make some progress.

The exercises and illustrations in this section are designed to help improve comprehension abilities. They include (1) Following Commands—nonverbal and verbal; (2) Pointing to objects, body parts, and pictures; (3) Use of gestures; (4) Use of a communication board.

FOLLOWING COMMANDS

Once it has been determined by testing that the patient has impaired comprehension, one should proceed by teaching him to follow commands, first nonverbal and then verbal. If the comprehension deficit is severe, start by teaching him to follow nonverbal commands, e.g. matching two like objects. In this exercise the patient is presented with common objects, i.e. a comb, key, and pencil. The clinician has a matching set. Without any verbal command, the clinician demonstrates matching items by holding up two like objects. For example, the clinician holds up a "key" and the patient is instructed by gestures to find the matching key by pointing to it with his hand. Repeated demonstration usually improves the patient's performance. This is considered to be the easiest task because it involves the use of only one receptive communication channel, namely the visual channel, and gives the patient a chance to be successful on a simple level.

If a patient is able to perform this task, then have him match two like pictures. Then if he can do this, have him match a real object to a picture.

Next, the patient should practice following verbal commands, e.g. "Close your eyes." This exercise is next in order of difficulty since this involves decoding of the spoken word. One should have the patient listen to the clinician as he gives commands in a normal tone of voice. The clinician should not shout at the patient if he does not seem to understand but rather speak slowly. Shouting is not only ineffective but inappropriate. The patient's difficulty is a lack of understanding not an inability to hear what is being said. If the patient is unable to follow simple verbal commands, one should demonstrate the correct response simultaneously as he gives the spoken command. Then repeat the command without the demonstration and wait for the patient's response. This method will usually be helpful.

POINTING TO OBJECTS, BODY PARTS, AND PICTURES

After the patient is able to perform nonverbal matching tasks and is able to follow verbal commands, the next step is to teach the patient to point to objects named by the clinician. This is the next most difficult task since it involves decoding of the two receiving channels, namely, visual and auditory. The patient is presented with a few simple objects. While he looks at them (visual), he listens to the words (auditory) as the name of the object is spoken by the clinician. He is instructed to point to the item. For example. "Point to the cup," "Point to the spoon." When a patient is able to point to common objects named by the clinician, pictures of those objects are introduced—since this is slightly more difficult than pointing to a tangible object. The procedure is repeated, that is, the patient is shown a few simple pictures and is told to point to the picture as the name of the illustration is spoken by the clinician. Associating words to pictures aids in recall of language and vocabulary. The illustrations in this section are designed for this purpose. Begin with three pictures on a page. Have the patient point to the picture as the name of the picture is spoken. When the patient can select one item from three on a page, graduate him up to selecting one item from four, five, and six items on a page. This task is more difficult due to the increased number of visual stimuli and the increased range of possible choices.

Next, continue using the same pictures and vary the directions slightly, e.g. "Show me the cup," "Put your finger on the cup," "Touch the cup," "Where is the cup?" In this task only one variable, namely, the directional message, is altered while the pictures remain constant. In this way the difficuty of the task is increased in small steps. When a patient can respond correctly, the next step is to reduce the length of the directional message to one word, e.g. "cup, spoon, comb," etc. The clinician says only the key word and the patient is taught to point to the pictures named by the clinician. This is a more difficult task since the patient has less time to process the information and to decode the incoming message.

USE OF GESTURES

In many patients, the use of gesture language, in addition to speech, is impaired following a stroke or other brain injury. For the patient who cannot express himself verbally, especially in the beginning stages, it is important to teach the patient how to use gestures effectively. Very often a patient may nod his head "yes" when he means "no" without realizing that he is gesturing incorrectly. This results in frustration on both the part of the patient and his family members. Therefore, teaching a patient to nod his head appropriately to indicate "yes" and "no" may serve as an important tool for him in his attempts at communication and may provide the family with a means to understand the patient's basic needs. It is recommended that the family simplify matters by asking the patient simple concrete questions, e.g. "Do you want coffee?" Wait for the patient to nod his head, rather than asking "Do you want coffee or tea, now or later?" Asking one simply stated question at a time is easier for the patient to absorb.

USE OF A COMMUNICATION BOARD

In addition, for the nonverval patient who can understand the spoken word and can also understand simple written words, it is suggested that he be taught to use a "communication board" to express his basic needs. Simple everyday words are printed in a legible manner on a piece of cardboard paper or on a box. The patient is instructed to point to the appropriate word to indicate his basic needs and desires; for example, "I want_____" (water, tissue, doctor, bedpan, etc.) This method is used as a temporary alternative to oral expression of ideas. Once the patient can repeat and name items, he is encouraged to respond verbally as much as possible. In the meantime, however, the communication board can be an important useful aid to early communication attempts.

FOLLOW THESE DIRECTIONS:

Directions: Say these commands slowly to the patient. (If he cannot follow the directions, demonstrate the correct response.)

1. Close your eyes.

2. Raise your hand.

3. Put your hand on your chest.

4. Shake your head "yes."

5. Point to your nose.

6. Shake your head "no."

7. Point to the ceiling.

8. Point to the floor.

9. Open your mouth.

10. Stick out your tongue.

11. Turn your head to the right.

12. Turn your head to the left.

FOLLOW THESE DIRECTIONS:

Directions: Say these commands slowly to the patient.

1. Put your hand on your nose.

2. Stick out your tongue.

3. Close your eyes.

4. Open your mouth.

5. Raise your hand.

6. Point to the door.

7. Touch your hair.

8. Touch your mouth.

FOLLOWING COMMANDS

Directions: Have patient point to items in room.

Say:

1. **Point to the bed.**

2. **Point to the chair.**

3. **Point to the table.**

4. **Point to the window.**

5. **Point to the door.**

6. **Point to the closet.**

7. **Point to the bathroom.**

8. **Point to the light.**

9. **Point to the phone.**

10. **Point to the TV.**

11. **Point to the floor.**

12. **Point to the ceiling.**

13. **Point to the mirror.**

FOLLOWING COMMANDS

Directions: Have patient point to body parts.

Say:
1. **Point to your nose.**

2. **Point to your eyes.**

3. **Point to your mouth.**

4. **Point to your hair.**

5. **Point to your teeth.**

6. **Point to your chest.**

7. **Point to your ears.**

8. **Point to your neck.**

9. **Point to your shoulders.**

10. **Point to your feet.**

FOLLOWING COMMANDS

Directions: When the patient can point to body parts, have him listen to a clue and point to the body part spoken about.

Say:

1. **Point to something that you smell with.**

2. **Point to something that you hear with.**

3. **Point to something you stand on.**

4. **Point to something you see with.**

5. **Point to something you carry packages with.**

6. **Point to something you walk with.**

7. **Point to something you comb.**

8. **Point to something you clap with.**

9. **Point to something you listen with.**

10. **Point to something you walk with.**

FOLLOWING TWO—STAGE COMMANDS

Directions: Say these commands at a normal rate. (If the patient does not understand, repeat each command slowly. If he still doesn't understand, demonstrate the correct response after the command and wait for his response.)

1. **Point to your nose—then put your hand on your chest.**

2. **Point to the ceiling—then point to the floor.**

3. **Open your mouth and stick out your tongue.**

4. **Close your eyes—then raise your arm.**

5. **Put your hand on your shoulder—then put your hand on your knee.**

6. **Point to the window—then point to the door.**

7. **Point to your ear—then point to your nose.**

8. **Raise your hand—open your mouth.**

FOLLOWING TWO—STAGE COMMANDS

Directions: Place a comb, pencil, and a tissue in front of patient and give these commands.

Say:

1. **Pick up the pencil and give it to me.**

2. **Pick up the comb and put it in your pocket.**

3. **Pick up the comb and give it to me.**

4. **Pick up the tissue and blow your nose.**

5. **Point to the pencil and point to the comb.**

6. **Pick up the tissue and put it in your pocket.**

7. **Pick up the tissue and give it to me.**

8. **Pick up the comb and comb your hair.**

9. **Pick up the pencil and put it on top of the tissue.**

10. **Pick up the pencil and put it next to the comb.**

POINTING TO PICTURES

Directions: Use the illustrations of body parts that follow this exercise (pages 19 to 21). Have the patient point to pictures as you name them.

<u>EYES</u>   <u>NOSE</u>   <u>MOUTH</u>

Say: **Point to the eyes.**

Point to the nose.

Point to the mouth.

<u>ARM</u>   <u>LEG</u>   <u>FEET</u>

Say: **Point to the arm.**

Point to the leg.

Point to the feet.

<u>EAR</u>   <u>HAIR</u>   <u>HANDS</u>

Say: **Point to the ear.**

Point to the hair.

Point to the hands.

(Then, present items in random order.)

BODY PARTS

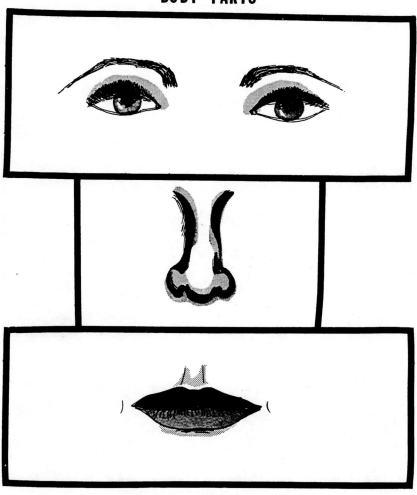

eyes   nose   mouth

BODY PARTS

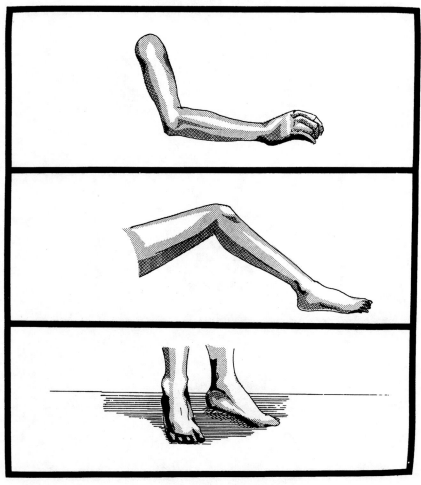

arm   leg   feet

BODY PARTS

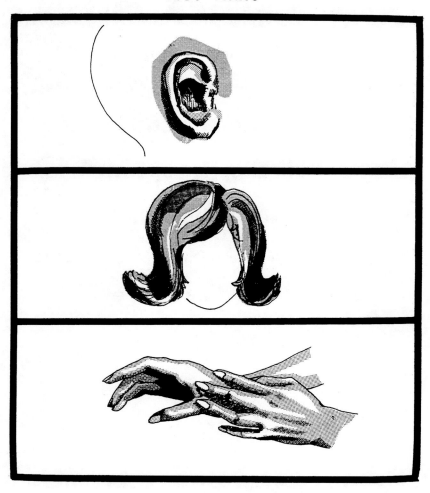

ear   hair   hands

POINTING TO PICTURES

Directions: Have the patient point to random object pictures as you name the illustrations on the following two pages. (If the patient doesn't seem to understand, vary the directions, i.e. say "Where is the cup?" or "Touch the cup," and demonstrate by pointing to the correct picture.)

Using the illustration that has three pictures on page 23,

Say: **Point to the cup.**

Point to the spoon.

Point to the pencil.

Using the illustration that has four pictures on page 24,

Say: **Point to the money.**

Point to the key.

Point to the glasses.

Point to the tissue.

(Then, present items in random order.)

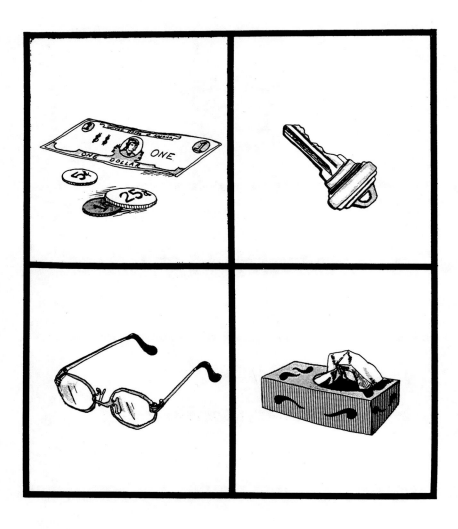

POINTING TO PICTURES

Directions: Have the patient point to random object pictures as you name the illustrations on the following pages. (If the patient doesn't seem to understand, vary the directions, i.e. say "Put your finger on the bed," or "Show me the bed," and demonstrate by pointing to the correct picture.)

Using the illustration that has five pictures on page 27,

Say: **Point to the bed.**

Point to the window.

Point to the door.

Point to the phone.

Point to the light.

Using the illustration that has six pictures on page 28,

Say: **Point to the pills.**

Point to the pen.

Point to the newspaper.

Point to the bell.

Point to the hanger.

Point to the shoes.

(Then, present items in random order.)

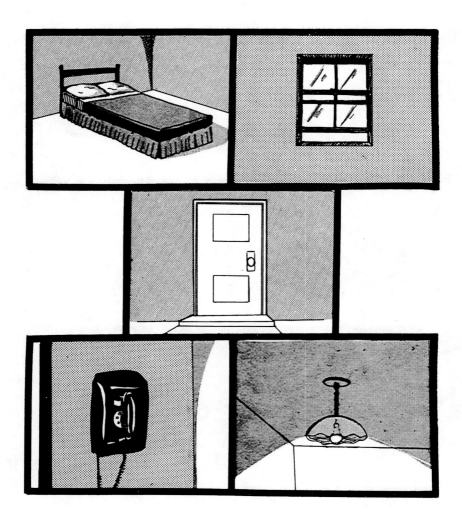

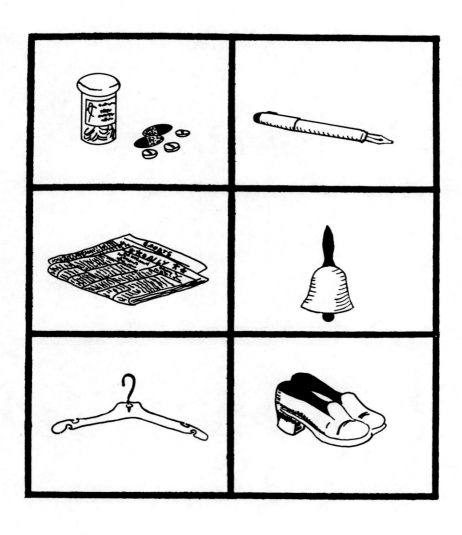

POINTING TO PICTURES

Directions: Have patient point to pictures as you name them.

(For additional pratice in picture recognition and to help improve comprehension of the spoken word, use the illustrations of useful objects in categories that are included in Section Three of this manual, on pages 182 to 207.)

Pictures of useful items have been arranged in categories as listed below. Begin with the category, Grooming, and say— "Point to the comb, Point to the brush," etc. Repeat this procedure for all pictures.

grooming

clothing

food

drink

furniture

tableware

household items

appliances

entertainment

transportation

up and down

tools

GESTURING "YES" AND "NO"

Directions: The patient shakes his head "yes" or "no" as the clinician points to random object pictures and asks these questions. (Use the illustrations on the preceding pages.)

Using the illustration that has three pictures on page 23,

Say: **Is this a cup?**

Is this a spoon?

Is this a pencil?

Using the illustration that has four pictures on page 24,

Say: **Is this some money?**

Is this a key?

Is this a pair of glasses?

Is this a box of tissues?

(Then, present items in random order.)

GESTURING "YES" AND "NO"

Directions: The patient shakes his head "yes" or "no" as the clinician points to random object pictures and asks these questions. (Use the illustrations on the preceding pages.)

Using the illustration that has five pictures on page 27,

Say: **Is this a bed?**

Is this a window?

Is this a door?

Is this a phone?

Is this a light?

Using the illustration that has six pictures on page 28,

Say: **Is this a bottle of pills?**

Is this a pen?

Is this a newspaper?

Is this a bell?

Is this a hanger?

Is this a pair of shoes?

(Then, present items in random order.)

COMPREHENSION OF "YES" AND "NO" AND NODDING CORRECTLY

Directions: Ask the patient simple questions—have him shake his head to indicate his answer. (Help the patient by demonstrating the correct nod of head for each answer. Then repeat question and have him respond on his own.)

Say: Are all men tall? *Patient's Response:*

(nod head)   yes or no

Are you a man?

Is your name John? (Use patient's real name)

Is the light on?

Did you eat breakfast?

Is it daytime?

Are you in the hospital?

Are you thirsty?

Do you wear a dress?

Is your husband's name Jack? (Use real name)

Are you a woman?

Is your doctor's name
Dr. _____?
(Use correct name of physician)

Do apples grow on trees?

Does money grow on trees?

Is it cold in winter?

Is it cold in summer?

Are you at home now?

Are you standing up?

Are you sitting in a chair?

Are you in bed now?

Is the television on now?

Are all women short?

Do cats fly?

Do birds fly?

SHAKE YOUR HEAD "YES" AND "NO"

Directions: Ask these questions and have patient respond by nodding his head appropriately.

Say:
1. Are you tired?

2. Are you thirsty?

3. Are you cold?

4. Are you hungry?

5. Are you sleepy?

6. Do you want water?

7. Do you have pain?

8. Do you want the bedpan?

9. Do you want the nurse?

10. Do you want to eat?

USE OF GESTURES AND A COMMUNICATION BOARD

For patients who cannot communicate verbally but who can understand spoken and written language, the use of a "communication board" is suggested. Especially in the beginning it is extremely important that the patient be talked to and be encouraged to convey his basic desires and feelings in a simple nonverbal way. A piece of strudy paper or a cardboard box can be used as a communication board. On it, in large legible writing, one should put the patient's name and the names of the patient's close family members and items of special interest; for example, wife's name, son's name, daughter's name, grandchildren's names, doctor's name, names of close friends, etc. Put the words "yes" and "no" in large capitals so that the patient may point to these words to answer questions.

Also record the patient's feelings, e.g. *I feel*

cold	**tired**	**depressed**
hot	**angry**	**okay**
hungry	**sick**	**wet**
dirty	**pain**	**nauseous**

Also record the patient's wants, e.g. *I want*

nurse	**urinal**	**bedpan**
water	**food**	**coffee**
doctor	**medicine**	**phone**

wife	husband	blanket
glasses	robe	slippers
tissue	shampoo	comb
TV	mirror	pillow

Also record the patient's wish, e.g. *I want to go*

| bathroom | home | outside |
| downstairs | wash | therapy |

Have the patient point to words to express his basic needs and feelings. In this way a patient is able to communicate on a limited scale in a nonverbal way.

POINT TO WORDS TO INDICATE WHAT YOU WANT

Directions: Write these words on a sturdy piece of paper. Have
patient point to them accordingly.

doctor	**nurse**
robe	**slippers**
glasses	**tissue**
water	**bathroom**
bedpan	**pills**
paper	**pencil**
yes	**no**

USE OF THE ALPHABET
FOR NONVERBAL COMMUNICATION

For patients who can match some words to pictures indicating that some residual reading comprehension ability is intact, it is suggested that a family member use several index cards cut into equal squares on which the letters of the alphabet should be printed in large, easy-to-read capitals. Felt-tip pen or crayon is suitable for this purpose. Make doubles of all the consonants and triples of the vowels, namely: A, E, I, O, U since these letters are often repeated in a single word. Any word requiring more than this amount can be accommodated by addition of the particular letter to the group on extra blank square cards. The ideal actual letter size should be approximately one-inch by one-inch.

When the alphabet letter set is completed, the patient is presented with the letters in his name. His name is repeated by the clinician—the patient listens and looks at the printed word even if he is unable to repeat it correctly. Then the clinician scrambles the letters and the patient is asked to arrange the letters in the proper order to spell his name. This procedure is repeated for many short useful words. In this way the patient is encouraged to respond and attempt to communicate in a nonverbal way. Even if the patient is unable to say the word aloud or to select the letters from the alphabet himself, just the ability to arrange the preselected letters into a meaningful word allows the patient to experience some degree of satisfaction in achieving mastery of this skill.

SECTION II

IMITATIVE ABILITY
AND ARTICULATION DRILLS

A) Strengthening the oral musculature tongue and lip exercises

B) Repetition practice—lists of words and sentences of increasing length

C) Articulation drills for individual consonant sounds

IMITATIVE ABILITY
AND ARTICULATION DRILLS

THE DRILLS IN THIS SECTION are designed to help patients who have difficulty imitating speech sounds due to weakness of the oral musculature, and to help those who have difficulty repeating speech sounds due to lack of voluntary control. Included are tongue and lip exercises designed to strengthen the oral musculature necessary for speech and word drills to improve repetition ability and defective articulation.

Strengthening the oral musculature and gaining voluntary control can be accomplished in steps: The first phase of strengthening the oral musculature is to practice imitation of gross oral movements such as opening and closing the mouth, protruding the tongue, moving it from side to side, raising and lowering the tongue-tip, rounding the lips, and smiling. It may be advantageous to have the patient practice in front of a large table mirror to help the patient gain more awareness of his oral movements. Practicing face-to-face is also recommended. Many patients actually prefer this method since it eliminates the embarrassment they feel in seeing their facial and lip disfigurement and sometimes drooling on the affected side. A tongue depressor used to indicate correct tongue and lip placement is also helpful.

When the imitation of oral movements is accomplished satisfactorily, one may proceed to the imitation of sounds. Some patients may be unable to make any sound at will although there is no vocal cord damage. Very often these patients are heard to cough or clear their throat involuntarily. These patients must be taught to phonate on command by beginning from reflexive sounds such as coughing, sighing while yawning, clearing the throat, or humming a familiar tune, to repetition of these acts on a voluntary basis. Specific exercises to encourage phonation have been included, e.g. have the patient feel your vocal cords vibrate, then press his hand to his neck and have him try to imitate making a sound.

After the patient is able to phonate, one may proceed to imitation of vowel sounds. When the patient can imitate the vowel sounds, he is then ready to advance to imitating short words. Begin with words that are useful and easy to see, e.g. "me," "more," "my," "bye," "bed," "back," "push," "please." Next, proceed to words with two syllables, e.g. "morning," "bye-bye," etc. When the patient can repeat words that begin with the same sound easily, have him repeat short words in ramdom order. Use the illustrations in Section Three for practice in repeating names of useful items. When the patient can accomplish this task, have him repeat words of increasing length, e.g. "help," "helpful," "helpfulness," etc. Lists of one, two, three, and four syllable words of increasing length are included, as well as sentences.

Many patients demonstrate dysarthria, resulting in slurred speech; therefore, articulation word drills to improve proper sound production have been included. They have been arranged to facilitate production, beginning with the easy-to-see lip sounds, i.e. "m," "p," "b," rather than in alphabetical order. Word lists of consonant sounds in the initial, medial, and final positions of words have been included, as well as some practice sentences emphasizing the sound. The words "make," "summer," and "home" and the sentence "What time are you coming home?" are samples of words and sentences stressing the consonant "m" sound.

The enterprising clinician or family member should improvise and add to these articulation drill-lists, words that specifically pertain to the patient's special interests, previous occupation, hobbies, and names of family members. A tape recording should be made of the patient's speech at the onset so that a comparison of progress can be made at intervals.

In addition to articulation disorders, e.g. sound distortions, substitutions, and omissions, the dysarthric patient may also demonstrate voice changes. His voice quality may become hypernasal or hoarse, etc., pitch may become abnormally low or high, rate may become abnormally slow or rapid. Exercises to improve voice quality have not been included but references on vocal rehabilitation are listed at the end of this manual under the heading "Suggested References," (see entry #7).

IMITATION OF GROSS ORAL MOVEMENTS

Directions: Have patient look in mirror or practice face-to-face while looking at clinician.

1. Have patient open and close mouth.

2. Have patient round lips.

3. Have patient round lips and try to throw a kiss.

4. Have patient smile.

5. Have patient protrude tongue.

6. Have patient protrude tongue and move it from side to side.

7. Have patient protrude tongue and lick upper lip.

8. Have patient protrude tongue and lick lower lip.

FACIAL EXERCISES
TO STRENGTHEN ORAL MUSCULATURE

Directions: Have patient imitate these oral movements while watching your mouth. (Repeat each item ten times, twice a day.)

1. **Open mouth wide—as if saying "ah," then round lips—as if saying "oo."**

2. **Round lips then smile.**

3. **Puff up cheeks. Hold air for five seconds—then release air as you blow out.**

4. **Suck in cheeks—then relax.**

5. **Open mouth wide—as if you're screaming—then relax.**

6. **Let lips flap—as you blow air out over them.**

7. **Puff up cheeks with air—move air from one cheek to the other without letting air escape lips. Alternate from one side to the other.**

LIP EXERCISES

Directions:　To strengthen weakened lip muscles, practice
each item ten times—twice a day.

1. **Round lips.**

2. **Smile.**

3. **Alternate rounding lips and smiling as if saying (oo)—(ee).**

4. **Open mouth wide—then round lips as if you are kissing.**

5. **Practice throwing a kiss.**

6. **Close lips tightly as if you are saying (mm).**

7. **Say ma ma ma ma (as fast as you can).**

8. **Say me me me me (as fast as you can).**

9. **Close lips tightly as you puff up your cheeks with air. Hold air inside cheeks for five seconds, then release.**

TONGUE EXERCISES

Directions: Watch the face of the clinician—imitate tongue movements.

1. **Protrude tongue—retract.**

2. **Move tongue from side to side.**

3. **Elevate tongue tip—point toward your nose.**

4. **Lower tongue top—point toward your chin.**

5. **Rotate tongue from side to side under upper lip while holding lips gently closed.**

6. **Repeat #5 on inside of lower lip.**

7. **Make a circle with tongue on inside of lips, holdings lips closed.**

Repeat as fast as you can—

la la la   **lucky lucky**

lee lee lee   **little lady**

lu lu lu   **hello hello hello**

lie down   **a little later**

ENCOURAGING PHONATION

Directions: Demonstrate making a sound—have patient imitate.

1. **Have patient cough—then try to say "ah."**

2. **Have patient yawn—then say "ah."**

3. **Have patient clear throat—then try to say "ah."**

4. **Pinch patient's nostrils tightly so that he is forced to breathe in through mouth—have him inhale and then exhale while saying "ah."**

5. **Tell patient to inhale deeply—then say "ah" while exhaling as if he is very exhausted.**

6. **Hold a telephone to his ear—have him try to say "hello."**

7. **Let patient feel your vocal cords vibrate as you say a sound. (Place his hand on your neck to feel the**

vibration.) Then have him try to imitate making a sound. Place his hand on his own neck to feel the vibration as he tries to say "ah."

8. Have the patient try to sing in unison with you. Hum a familiar tune and have him try to sing along.

9. Push in on the abdomen and apply hand pressure to the diaphragm as the patient exhales forcefully and tries to produce sound.

IMITATION OF VOWELS

Directions: When the patient can phonate consistently, say these vowels after the clinician.

1. **AH** (open mouth, breathe in, and exhale sighing) as in "h<u>o</u>t"

2. **OO** (round lips tightly) as in "t<u>oo</u>"

3. **EE** (smile as you raise sides of tongue) as in "m<u>e</u>"

4. **O** (round lips and open mouth slightly) as in "n<u>o</u>"

5. **OW** (open mouth wide, say "ae" as in "c<u>at</u>" and then round lips tightly for "oo") as in "n<u>ow</u>"

6. **I** (say "ah" then smile and say "ee"—combine for i-e) as in "p<u>ie</u>"

IMITATION OF AUTOMATIC SPEECH

Directions: When the patient can imitate vowels, have him imitate automatic speech expressions.

1. **Have the patient count in unison with you. Say the numbers 1, 2, 3, 4, 5—then have him try to say the numbers on his own.**

2. **Have him say the days of the week in unison with you— Monday, Tuesday, Wednesday, etc.—then have patient repeat on his own.**

3. **Have patient repeat his name.**

4. **Have him repeat other family member's names.**

5. **Have him repeat these short useful words:**

hi	up
bye	down
yes	no

now

hello

bye-bye

thank you

please

good

doctor

help

wait

REPETITION OF WORDS

Directions: The patient watches the lips of the clinician and
then tries to repeat each word. It may be necessary
to manipulate the patient's lips into the proper position to start the word. Begin practice with initial
sounds that are easy to see, e.g. lip sounds "m," "p,"
"b." Follow the order used in the articulation drills.
However, use only the lists of initial consonant
sounds, i.e. beginning sounds, until the patient can
repeat easily. The articulation drills begin on pages
77 to 123.

Repeat after the clinician:

me	bye	pay
my	bed	push
may	bath	pull
more	back	pick
much	big	please

When the patient can repeat single syllable words, try two syllable words and phrases:

maybe	bye-bye	push me
morning	be back	pull me
much more	bathroom	pay me

REPEATING WORDS IN RANDOM ORDER

Directions: When the patient is able to repeat words beginning with the same sounds easily, he is ready to begin repetition of words beginning with different sounds. Use the illustrations of useful items arranged in categories that are included in Section Three, pages 182 to 207. The clinician says the name of the picture and the patient repeats the words after him. The patient should be able to repeat most of the words correctly before attempting the more difficult task of naming the picture.

REPETITION OF NUMBERS

Directions: Listen to the clinician say each set of numbers, then repeat after him.

1—2

7—5

9—1—7

5—3—1

8—9—1—4

7—5—8—8

6—3—4—9—1

1—6—7—4—4

1—3—3—0—0—4

4—2—5—7—6—1

8—9—5—3—1—2—8

5—3—4—3—6—7—10

WORDS OF INCREASING LENGTH

Directions: Repeat these words after the clinician.

good	goodbye
thank	thank you
sun	sunshine
bath	bathroom
all	all right
pill	pillow
for	forgive
be	before
care	careful
to	today
win	window
more	morning

WORDS OF INCREASING LENGTH

Directions: Repeat these words after the clinician.

cup	cupcake
dough	donut
light	lightbulb
heart	heartbeat
life	lifeguard
hair	haircomb
count	countdown
card	cardroom
hand	handwash
base	basement
court	courtyard
hall	hallway

WORDS OF INCREASING LENGTH

Directions: Repeat these words after the clinician.

can	candy
den	dentist
rest	restroom
drug	drugstore
bath	bathroom
arm	armchair
door	doorstep
head	headstart
hard	hardware
short	shortcake
board	boardwalk
book	bookstore
cup	cupcake

WORDS OF INCREASING LENGTH

Directions: Repeat these words after the clinician.

foot	football
hot	hotdog
ear	eardrum
store	storeroom
play	playground
short	shortcut
up	upset
hang	hanger
on	onset
side	sidewalk
down	downtown
band	bandage

WORDS OF INCREASING LENGTH

Directions: Repeat these words after the clinician.

girl	girlfriend
heat	heatwave
pop	popcorn
land	landmark
hand	handmade
shirt	shirtwaist
some	someone
head	headstart
shop	shopworn
bed	bedspread
can	cannot
mess	message

WORDS OF INCREASING LENGTH

Directions: Repeat these words after the clinician.

pen	pencil
head	headache
down	downtown
pill	pillbox
tooth	toothache
pan	pancake
wrist	wristwatch
suit	suitcase
door	doorman
tea	teabag
day	daybreak
news	newsboy

WORDS OF INCREASING LENGTH

Directions: Repeat these words after the clinician.

flash	flashlight
off	office
car	carwash
card	cardboard
book	bookstore
clock	clockwise
land	landslide
corn	cornflakes
lip	lipstick
door	doorknob
but	butler
fruit	fruitstand
glass	glassware

WORDS OF INCREASING LENGTH

Directions: Repeat these words after the clinician.

news	newspaper
side	sidewalk
book	bookstore
land	landscape
look	lookout
cross	crosswalk
hot	hotdog
base	basement
time	timepiece
foot	football
down	downstairs
up	upstairs

WORDS OF INCREASING LENGTH

Directions: Repeat these words after the clinician.

apart	apartment
advise	adviser
subtract	subtraction
contract	contractor
instruct	instructor
inhale	inhalation
produce	production
expense	expensive
prescribe	prescription
describe	description
cancel	cancellation
recover	recovery

WORDS OF INCREASING LENGTH

Directions: Repeat these words after the clinician.

joy	joyful	joyfully
waste	wasteful	wastefully
clean	cleaning	cleanliness
joke	joking	jokingly
sweet	sweeten	sweetener
hope	hopeful	hopefully
wealth	wealthy	wealthier
sharp	sharpen	sharpener
weak	weaken	weakening
tease	teasing	teasingly
care	careful	carefully
sick	sicken	sickening

WORDS OF INCREASING LENGTH

Directions: Repeat these words after the clinician.

help	helpful	helpfulness
taste	tasty	tastier
fright	frighten	frightening
please	pleasing	pleasingly
force	forceful	forcefully
fool	foolish	foolishly
trick	tricky	trickery
long	longing	longingly
live	lively	livelihood
like	likely	likelihood
haste	hasty	hastily
aim	aimless	aimlessly

WORDS OF INCREASING LENGTH

Directions: Repeat these words after the clinician.

medicate	medication
organize	organization
condition	conditional
substitute	substitution
decorate	decoration
operate	operation
respectful	respectfully
photograph	photographer
institute	institution
visual	visualize
televise	television
obligate	obligation

WORDS OF INCREASING LENGTH

Directions: Repeat these words after the clinician.

physical	physical therapy
hospital	hospitalize
medical	medical center
transport	transportation
communicate	communication
speech	speech pathology
indicate	indication
medicine	medication
compatible	compatibility
associate	association
medicare	medicare office
compliment	complimentary

WORDS OF INCREASING LENGTH

Directions: Repeat these words after the clinician.

reason	reasoning	reasonable
drama	dramatic	dramatically
absorb	absorbent	absorbency
contract	contraction	contractual
music	musical	musically
decrease	decreasing	decreasingly
increase	increasing	increasingly
person	personal	personally
sincere	sincerely	sincerity
success	successful	successfully
forgive	forgiving	forgiveable
attract	attractive	attractiveness

MEMORY RETENTION
REPETITION PRACTICE

Directions: Listen to each sentence, then repeat it.

Sit down.

Sit down, please.

Thank you.

Thank you very much.

Thank you very much for every-thing.

Come in.

Come in, please.

Come in, please, and have a seat.

Come in, please, someone will help you right away.

So long.

So long, see you soon.

So long, it was so nice to see you.

MEMORY RETENTION
REPETITION PRACTICE

Directions: Listen to each sentence, then repeat it.

In the bathroom, there is a sink.

In the bathroom, there is a toilet.

In the bathroom, there is a tub.

In the bathroom, there is a sink, toilet, and tub.

In the office, there is a desk.

In the office, there is a chair.

In the office, there is a typewriter.

In the office, there is a desk, chair and typewriter.

**MEMORY RETENTION
REPETITION PRACTICE**

Directions: Listen to each sentence, then repeat it.

In the bedroom, there is a bed.

In the bedroom, there is a dresser.

In the bedroom, there is a night table.

In the bedroom, there is a lamp.

In the bedroom, there is a bed, dresser, night table, and lamp.

In the kitchen, there is a sink.

In the kitchen, there is a stove.

In the kitchen, there is a refrigerator.

In the kitchen, there is a dishwasher.

In the kitchen, there is a sink, stove, refrigerator, and dishwasher.

**MEMORY RETENTION
REPETITION PRACTICE**

Directions: Listen to each sentence, then repeat it.

In the hospital, there are doctors.

In the hospital, there are nurses.

In the hospital, there are patients.

In the hospital, there are doctors, nurses, and patients.

In the restaurant, there are customers.

In the restaurant, there are waiters.

In the restaurant, there is a cook.

In the restaurant, there is a cashier.

In the restaurant, there are waiters, customers, a cook, and a cashier.

MEMORY RETENTION
REPETITION PRACTICE

Directions: Listen to each sentence, then repeat it.

I like sports. I like golf, tennis, and swimming.

I like sports. I like football, baseball, and basketball.

I like holidays. I like Christmas, Thanksgiving, and New Year's Eve.

I like holidays. I like Easter, Labor Day, and the Fourth of July.

I like cars. I like Buick, Chrysler, and Cadillac.

I like sports cars. I like Mercedes, Rolls Royce, and Jaguar.

I like foods. I like meat, cheese, and eggs.

I like foods. I like steak, chicken, and fish.

REPETITION PRACTICE

Directions: Listen to each sentence, then repeat it.

I like fruits.

I like apples, oranges, and pears.

I like bananas, grapes, and plums.

I like vegetables.

I like peas, corn, and beans.

I like spinach, broccoli, and cau-liflower.

I like desserts.

I like pie, cake, and ice cream.

I like jello, fruit, and pudding.

I drink.

I drink water, juice, and coffee.

I drink milk, tea, and liquor.

I wear clothing.

I wear shoes, socks, and a belt.

I wear a shirt, pants, and a tie (for a man).

I wear a dress, skirt, and a blouse (for a woman).

ARTICULATION DRILL
"M" SOUND

Directions: Press lips together and hum "mm."

make	summer	home
more	hamburger	come
made	timetable	room
morning	stomach	same
money	something	some
many	sometime	name
much	roomy	shame
Monday	roommate	dime
move	timing	ham
match	coming	time

How <u>m</u>uch is it?

I want so<u>me</u> <u>m</u>ore.

Do you have a di<u>me</u>?

Good <u>m</u>orning!

What ti<u>me</u> are you co<u>m</u>ing ho<u>me</u>?

So<u>me</u> things see<u>m</u> the sa<u>me</u>.

<u>M</u>illions of <u>m</u>en were <u>m</u>arching.

The <u>m</u>eeting is on <u>M</u>onday <u>m</u>orning.

<u>M</u>artha <u>m</u>akes <u>m</u>any things.

How <u>m</u>uch <u>m</u>ore <u>m</u>oney can I <u>m</u>ake?

<u>M</u>embers of <u>m</u>y fa<u>m</u>ily are <u>m</u>eeting.

ARTICULATION DRILL
"P" SOUND

Directions: Close lips, puff up cheeks, and then let air explode as you say "p."

pie	paper	cup
piece	people	top
pay	happy	tip
pen	napkin	soap
push	apple	soup
pull	happen	sip
pills	supper	wipe
pin	proper	rope
pencil	open	lap
please	upper	nap

Get me the newspaper.

I like apple pie.

Give me a pencil and paper.

Pardon me, please.

Pull up a chair.

He broke the zipper on his pants.

For supper they had fresh snapper.

Can you pick a ripe pineapple?

She prepared a delicious supper.

Buy me some peanuts and popcorn.

Wash up with soap and water.

ARTICULATION DRILL
"B" SOUND

Directions: Press lips together—puff up cheeks with air—let air explode as vocal cords vibrate and you say "buh."

bye	**maybe**	**rub**
bed	**baby**	**cab**
better	**table**	**bib**
bedpan	**able**	**Bob**
bad	**trouble**	**knob**
box	**ribbon**	**rib**
before	**garbage**	**fib**
back	**cabbage**	**gab**
because	**ruby**	**tub**
bathroom	**elbow**	**sub**

I need the <u>b</u>edpan.

I want to get <u>b</u>etter.

My <u>b</u>ack hurts.

I want to go to the <u>b</u>athroom.

Good-<u>b</u>ye!

Pick up the <u>b</u>a<u>b</u>y.

Come <u>b</u>ack <u>b</u>efore noon.

<u>B</u>athe in the <u>b</u>athtu<u>b</u>.

<u>B</u>ring me my ro<u>b</u>e.

Put the <u>b</u>ox on the ta<u>b</u>le.

I eat <u>b</u>read and <u>b</u>utter.

<u>B</u>ill helped take out the gar<u>b</u>age.

The <u>b</u>oys liked to go to the <u>b</u>each.

ARTICULATION DRILL
"W" SOUND

Directions: Round lips in a small circle as if you were saying the sound "oo."

way	awake	how
won	away	window
wake	showing	know
we	snowing	show
wait	going	go
will	sewing	low
water	doing	toe
week	knowing	knew
want	lower	shoe
was	flower	chew

Lower the window please.

Please wake me up.

What are you doing?

Where and when shall I meet you?

Which way are you going?

Wait until next week.

Will you meet me at one?

I want some water.

I wonder how it will work out.

It's good to know how.

When she received the flowers she was happy.

Walter went out to take a walk.

ARTICULATION DRILL
"F" SOUND

Directions: Put upper front teeth over lower lip—blow air
gently out over lip as you say "f."

f̲ine	cof̲fee	wif̲e
f̲our	ef̲fort	laug̲h̲
f̲ive	of̲fer	coug̲h̲
f̲ast	waf̲er	roug̲h̲
f̲irst	of̲ten	half̲
F̲riday	af̲ter	knif̲e
f̲eet	saf̲er	cuf̲f̲
f̲ood	sof̲a	toug̲h̲
f̲ind	coug̲h̲ing	enoug̲h̲
f̲uss	laug̲h̲ing	stuf̲f̲

I <u>f</u>eel <u>f</u>ine.

See you on <u>F</u>riday.

I have a cou<u>gh</u>.

Bring me some <u>f</u>ood.

I like co<u>ff</u>ee.

Do you like <u>f</u>resh or <u>f</u>rozen vegetables?

<u>F</u>ind the <u>f</u>ront door key.

Walk as <u>f</u>ast as you can.

Don't <u>f</u>orget to buy the <u>f</u>ood.

Keep some <u>f</u>ood in the <u>f</u>reezer.

How o<u>f</u>ten do you shop <u>f</u>or <u>f</u>ood?

Do you drink co<u>ff</u>ee <u>f</u>or break<u>f</u>ast?

ARTICULATION DRILL
"V" SOUND

Directions: Put top front teeth over bottom lip—blow air out gently as your vocal cords vibrate and you say "vuh."

very	even	love
vest	oven	stove
visit	every	dive
voice	driven	live
vacation	never	weave
victory	driver	sleeve
victim	proven	cave
vase	river	have
vial	ever	heave
value	evil	leave

I haven't seen Dave lately.

My voice is hoarse.

Turn off the stove.

When are you leaving?

When is your vacation?

Your advice was very good.

Our vacation was very expensive.

Vested suits are in vogue.

Gold prices vary every day.

The value of the vase was never determined.

He took an overdose of Valium®.

Everyone's values are different. It is up to the individual.

ARTICULATION DRILL
VOICELESS "TH" SOUND

Directions: Stick tongue out between teeth—blow air out gently as you say "th."

think	birthday	with
thumb	anything	breath
thousand	nothing	both
thirteen	something	bath
thought	bathtub	north
thirsty	Martha	worth
thigh	author	earth
thanks	worthwhile	mouth
thirty	Arthur	south
three	leather	math

Happy bir<u>th</u>day!

What do you <u>th</u>ink?

I will <u>th</u>ink it over.

Bo<u>th</u> of us are <u>th</u>irsty.

<u>Th</u>ank you very much!

Where is the ba<u>th</u>room?

Ar<u>th</u>ur <u>th</u>inks this book is wor<u>th</u>-while.

What mon<u>th</u> is your bir<u>th</u>day?

<u>Th</u>anks for <u>th</u>e bir<u>th</u>day present.

The lea<u>th</u>er jacket is wor<u>th</u> a lot of money.

You can see your brea<u>th</u> in the cold wea<u>th</u>er.

They won <u>th</u>ree <u>th</u>ousand dollars in the contes<u>t</u>.

Some<u>th</u>ing is better than no<u>th</u>ing.

ARTICULATION DRILL
VOICED "TH" SOUND

Directions: Stick tongue out between teeth and blow air out gently as vocal cords vibrate as you say "thuh."

the	other	breathe
this	brother	loathe
that	another	bathe
then	mother	clothe
those	father	with
they	clothing	
their	leather	
them	bathing	
than	together	
these	weather	

Is the clothing made of leather?

Those are yours, these are mine.

I can hardly breathe.

Give me another.

Do you want this one or that one?

They got together on their birth-days.

They got new clothes for the party.

Their mother and father were proud of them.

The bathing suit came with a matching shirt.

They owned a clothing store.

The hot weather was bothersome.

ARTICULATION DRILL
"T" SOUND

Directions: Place tongue up behind front teeth—let air pressure explode as tongue tip is lowered and you say "t."

take	better	hot
time	hotter	not
touch	letter	what
tell	sweater	hurt
talk	heater	wait
teeth	enter	late
table	eating	tight
tomorrow	bottles	tonight
today	seating	closet
teach	getting	light

Please don'<u>t</u> come la<u>te</u>.

I<u>t</u>'s ge<u>tt</u>ing <u>t</u>oo la<u>te</u>.

I mus<u>t</u> <u>t</u>ake my pills.

<u>T</u>urn ou<u>t</u> the ligh<u>t</u>.

See you <u>t</u>onigh<u>t</u>.

I wan<u>t</u> <u>t</u>ea and <u>t</u>oast.

<u>T</u>ake your <u>t</u>ime.

<u>T</u>ake my <u>t</u>emperature.

The <u>t</u>ables are <u>t</u>urned.

<u>T</u>urn off the <u>t</u>elevision.

I<u>t</u> is <u>t</u>oo ho<u>t</u> ou<u>t</u>side <u>t</u>oday.

Only <u>t</u>ime will <u>t</u>ell.

<u>T</u>ell me the <u>t</u>rue s<u>t</u>ory.

Wha<u>t</u> do you wan<u>t</u>?

Will you please wai<u>t</u> a minu<u>te</u>?

ARTICULATION DRILL
"D" SOUND

Directions: Put your tongue up behind upper front teeth—
let vocal cords vibrate as you say "duh,"

do	daddy	bad
don't	ready	bed
door	adding	food
doctor	loading	need
day	ladder	read
done	bladder	ride
down	scalding	side
dear	folding	wide
diet	reading	lend
dizzy	riding	made

Call the <u>d</u>octor.

I feel <u>d</u>izzy to<u>d</u>ay.

I'm on a <u>d</u>iet.

Open the <u>d</u>oor wi<u>d</u>e.

<u>D</u>on't <u>d</u>o it.

<u>D</u>o me a favor.

Are you rea<u>d</u>y to go <u>d</u>owntown?

<u>D</u>on't stay in be<u>d</u> all <u>d</u>ay.

<u>D</u>o you rea<u>d</u> the <u>d</u>aily paper?

<u>D</u>o you spen<u>d</u> much time in the <u>d</u>en?

<u>D</u>o you nee<u>d</u> more foo<u>d</u>?

He ha<u>d</u> <u>d</u>ifficulty seeing to the right si<u>d</u>e.

ARTICULATION DRILL
"N" SOUND

Directions: Put tongue up behind upper front teeth—let air come through nose. Make vocal cords vibrate as you say "en."

no	honey	run
now	funny	man
not	any	sun
never	many	fun
noisy	candy	one
name	money	cane
near	running	line
nice	sunny	fine
night	lining	sign
noon	finer	thin

<u>N</u>ot <u>n</u>ow, <u>n</u>ever!

I do<u>n</u>'t k<u>n</u>ow your <u>n</u>ame.

It's too <u>n</u>oisy.

Good <u>n</u>ight!

I said, <u>n</u>o!

<u>N</u>o o<u>n</u>e thought it was fu<u>nn</u>y.

Ca<u>n</u> you read the fi<u>ne</u> pri<u>nt</u> o<u>n</u> the sig<u>n</u>?

Sig<u>n</u> o<u>n</u> the dotted li<u>ne</u>.

Her li<u>ne</u> was co<u>n</u>sta<u>nt</u>ly busy.

The young ma<u>n</u> made lots of mo<u>ne</u>y.

Ca<u>n</u> you walk a straight li<u>ne</u>?

The moo<u>n</u> is full to<u>n</u>ight.

ARTICULATION DRILL
"L" SOUND

Directions: Place tongue up behind upper front teeth as you
say "la."

leave	alone	ball
late	lively	all
lady	lonely	call
later	lovely	small
let	only	tall
last	along	final
laugh	below	well
live	belong	will
lie	yellow	wall
lazy	jello	hall

Yes, I will call.

I hope I get well.

See you later.

I feel lonely.

Leave me alone!

Tell me your final decision.

Does this letter belong to you?

I believe I will get well.

This style looks well on you.

She is a tall beautiful girl.

Don't live a lazy life.

He learned his lesson well.

ARTICULATION DRILL
"L" BLENDS

Directions: Combine the consonants "P," "B" and "F" with the "L" sound as you say the words:

p l	b l	f l
please	blue	fly
place	blanket	flu
plaid	blame	flat
plus	blow	flirt
pleated	blurred	flavor
pleasure	black	fluffy
supply	bleeding	flight
reply	blink	floor
replace	blender	flush

He was <u>bl</u>ack and <u>bl</u>ue from the fall.

<u>Fl</u>ush the toilet.

What <u>fl</u>avor do you like best?

<u>Pl</u>ease re<u>pl</u>ace the light bulb.

She wore a pretty <u>bl</u>ouse.

The solution is com<u>pl</u>icated.

The <u>pl</u>umber re<u>pl</u>aced the broken pipe.

The priest gave the <u>bl</u>essing.

The com<u>pl</u>iment gave him a lot of <u>pl</u>easure.

<u>Pl</u>ease bring me another <u>bl</u>anket.

The college issued him a di<u>pl</u>oma.

The <u>fl</u>oor was too slippery.

ARTICULATION DRILL
"L" BLENDS CONTINUED

Directions: Combine the consonants "K," "G," and "S" with the "L" sound as you say these words:

k l	g l	sl
clean	gloves	slow
closet	glad	slip
clear	gloomy	sly
close	glamour	slur
claim	Gladys	slam
clap	glare	slim
clip	glue	slippers
cloudy	glow	slang
include	glass	slot
clock	glimpse	slit

I'm so <u>gl</u>ad you could come!

Take your <u>cl</u>othes to the <u>cl</u>eaners.

<u>Gl</u>oria is very <u>gl</u>amourous.

I need some <u>gl</u>ue.

She put her <u>cl</u>othes in the <u>cl</u>oset.

The girl was <u>sl</u>y and <u>cl</u>ever.

Can you see the <u>cl</u>ock <u>cl</u>early?

I must speak <u>sl</u>owly and <u>cl</u>early.

<u>Cl</u>ose the <u>cl</u>oset door.

She left her <u>sl</u>ippers on the floor.

Don't <u>sl</u>am the <u>cl</u>oset door.

ARTICULATION DRILL
"R" SOUND

Directions: Round lips slightly, open jaws slightly, curl tongue tip slightly backward as you say "er."

right	**carry**	**fire**
real	**hurry**	**tire**
really	**borrow**	**chair**
ready	**carrot**	**hair**
ring	**worry**	**store**
reason	**story**	**floor**
roll	**sorry**	**more**
rub	**nurse**	**color**
round	**purse**	**fair**
room	**worse**	**care**

My right arm hurts.

Am I right or wrong?

Don't worry, you can have more.

What is your phone number?

Call the nurse.

Tell me your version of the story.

I need to borrow more money.

The store caught on fire.

What is the real reason?

Hurry up, I'm in a rush.

I am sorry to hear about your mis-
fortune.

ARTICULATION DRILL
"R" BLENDS—"PR"—"TR"

Directions: Combine the consonants "P" and "T" with the "R" sound as you say these words:

pretty	**trap**
promise	**trouble**
pray	**trust**
practice	**treat**
predict	**try**
produce	**trip**
appreciate	**track**
compromise	**truth**
approximately	**trousers**
improvement	**truck**

Pray for me.

Practice makes perfect.

I appreciate your kindness.

I trust in you.

I hope I improve.

The nurse carried the medicine tray.

I will practice my lesson.

Tell me the trouble.

Which trousers should I take on the trip?

Trim the trees in the spring.

The train fell off the track.

ARTICULATION DRILL
"S" SOUND

Directions: Lips are smiling as you close teeth lightly and raise tongue tip and blow air out gently down center of mouth as you say "ss."

say	beside	house
so	inside	nice
sorry	outside	dress
sue	aside	ice
soap	grocer	mess
soup	saucer	twice
sign	faucet	police
see	dresser	office
sip	sister	lease
soda	mister	space

See you soon.

Clean up this mess.

Call your office.

Come inside and sit down.

I am so sorry.

The sink is stopped up.

Stay at my place.

Put the sofa in storage.

Buy some stocks and bonds.

Stop staring into space.

Study your speech lesson.

There is grass outside the house.

ARTICULATION DRILL
"Z" SOUND

Directions: Lips are smiling, teeth are lightly closed, tongue is up behind teeth as you blow air out gently and let vocal cords vibrate as you say "zzz."

zero	easy	please
zone	lazy	ease
zip	crazy	fees
zoo	razor	sneeze
zing	dozen	has
zigzag	reason	is
zipper	busy	nose
zebra	cousin	because

Please do these things for me.

Close your zipper.

What's your zip code?

I have to sneeze.

I shave with a razor.

ARTICULATION DRILL
"SH" SOUND

Directions: Round lips, raise sides of tongue to upper teeth, blow air out center of mouth as you say "sh."

shoe	washing	wash
shop	machine	wish
sure	dishes	cash
sugar	tissue	rash
sharp	ocean	rush
shave	issue	push
shelf	station	polish
sherbet	correction	dish
shine	direction	danish
share	option	finish

I love milkshakes and sherbets.

Be sure to send my best wishes.

Put the clothes in the washing machine.

I like to go fishing.

Put the dishes in the dishwasher.

Should I or shouldn't I go?

She has a sharp tongue.

Do you want to share the fish?

Put the shoes on the shelf.

Do your shoes match your shirt?

Where do you shop for shoes?

When will the wash be finished?

ARTICULATION DRILL
"CH" SOUND

Directions: Raise sides of tongue, round lips, explode air as
you combine "t" and "sh" sounds and say "ch."

check	teacher	each
checkbook	pitcher	watch
charge	watching	itch
chest	reaching	catch
church	itching	pinch
chief	departure	reach
cherry	bachelor	touch
cheese	feature	such
change	picture	much
cheat	stretcher	which

I need my <u>ch</u>eckbook.

I need my wristwat<u>ch</u>.

I have a pic<u>tu</u>re of my grand-<u>ch</u>ildren.

I can't rea<u>ch</u> him by phone.

Where is my <u>ch</u>arge plate?

<u>Ch</u>eck your depar<u>tu</u>re time.

Keep in tou<u>ch</u> with the tea<u>ch</u>er.

Whi<u>ch</u> pic<u>tu</u>re do you prefer?

We liked the <u>ch</u>eese very mu<u>ch</u>.

What is the fea<u>tu</u>re pic<u>tu</u>re?

The pit<u>ch</u>er threw the ball to the cat<u>ch</u>er.

ARTICULATION DRILL
"J" SOUND

Directions: Round lips—raise tongue tip to alveolar ridge—combine "d" and "zh" sound while vocal cords vibrate as you say "juh."

juice	**budget**	**edge**
just	**angel**	**orange**
jaw	**injure**	**ledge**
jury	**object**	**fudge**
jam	**badger**	**badge** .
judge	**conjure**	**bandage**
jelly	**ledger**	**coverage**
jiffy	**wages**	**footage**
jog	**pages**	**wage**
jar	**major**	**cage**

Do you like jam or jelly?

You can't be both judge and jury.

I like orange juice for breakfast.

A forger usually lands in jail.

Did you get injured on the job?

The jury deliberated the decision.

The jar of jam is on the shelf.

What coverage do you have for the injury?

The judge objected to the question.

The ledger pages are neat.

He injured himself jogging.

ARTICULATION DRILL
"K" SOUND

Directions: Raise back of tongue, let air explode as you say "k."

key	okay	cake
keep	making	make
kind	taking	take
kitchen	baking	bake
catch	faking	book
cut	lacking	look
cup	looking	pick
car	cookies	work
call	pocket	awake
cold	stockings	steak

He caught a cold.

He came by car.

It's okay with me.

Give me the car keys.

Can you call me later?

Keep my coffee hot.

He bought some cookies and cake.

Start the car with a key.

Did you come by car?

What are you baking in the kitchen?

Look in your pocket for the key.

Wake up on time for work.

ARTICULATION DRILL
"G" SOUND

Directions: Raise back of tongue, let air explode as vocal cords vibrate and you say "guh."

go	**begin**	**egg**
get	**began**	**leg**
give	**foggy**	**wig**
good	**soggy**	**fog**
gums	**beggar**	**rag**
gift	**nagging**	**bag**
game	**sagging**	**stag**
guess	**forgive**	**tag**
girl	**forget**	**sag**
guest	**jogging**	**nag**

Can you guess?

She got a card from the grandchildren.

Be my guest.

Go and get it.

Give it to me.

He broke his leg in the game.

The girl gave him a gift.

She begged him to forgive her.

It began to get foggy.

She gave her word to stop nagging.

She forgot to get the eggs.

The jogger broke his leg.

ARTICULATION DRILL
"H" SOUND

Directions: Open mouth, inhale and exhale as if panting as you say "h."

<u>h</u>ow	in<u>h</u>ale
<u>h</u>urry	ex<u>h</u>ale
<u>h</u>appy	ma<u>h</u>ogany
<u>h</u>usband	dis<u>h</u>earten
<u>h</u>urt	disin<u>h</u>erit
<u>h</u>is	pro<u>h</u>ibit
<u>h</u>ers	<u>h</u>ap<u>h</u>azard
<u>h</u>and	compre<u>h</u>end
<u>h</u>eart	fool<u>h</u>ardy
<u>h</u>am	post<u>h</u>aste

I am in a <u>h</u>urry.

I <u>h</u>ope to get better.

What's <u>h</u>appening in <u>h</u>ere?

Where is my <u>h</u>usband?

<u>H</u>ow about it?

Tell <u>h</u>im where it <u>h</u>urts.

<u>H</u>er <u>h</u>usband <u>h</u>urt <u>h</u>is back.

<u>H</u>e <u>h</u>ad a <u>h</u>appy marriage.

<u>H</u>urry over to my <u>h</u>ouse.

It is <u>h</u>ard to compre<u>h</u>end.

<u>H</u>e in<u>h</u>erited one <u>h</u>undred thousand dollars.

<u>H</u>ow did <u>h</u>e <u>h</u>urt <u>h</u>is <u>h</u>and?

VOCABULARY RECALL, GRAMMAR AND SYNTAX

A) Fill-in tasks and sentence completion

B) Illustrated useful objects in categories

C) Grammar usage and proper word order drills

D) Advanced fill-in sentences in paragraphs

VOCABULARY RECALL, GRAMMAR AND SYNTAX

SECTION THREE addresses itself to language impairments characterized by a reduction of available vocabulary and errors of grammar and syntax. This section includes exercises and illustrations which are designed to increase vocabulary and word recall skills. The exercises progress from simple to more complex material. First, begin with drills on opposites; e.g. you say "hot," have the patient say "cold." This is the simplest task because it involves automatic speech. Next, have the patient name things that go together, e.g. "table" and "chair."

Then, fill-in exercises of increasing difficulty have been provided. To begin, have patient fill in missing words to complete a phase, e.g. "a loaf of *bread*," "a glass of *water*," etc. Next, have him fill in appropriate words to complete a short sentence, e.g. "I wash with soap and *water*," "I eat bread and *butter*," etc. Read the beginning of the sentence aloud and have the patient finish the sentence in his own words. For the patient who is able to read aloud, have him read the entire exercise orally on his own and have him try to supply the correct response. There is no arbitrary correct answer. Any word that makes sense is acceptable; e.g. in the sentence "I drink a cup of _____," the words "coffee," "tea," "milk," or "water" are appropriate. Before beginning each exercise the clinician should give the patient several correct examples. A sample of the correct response has been provided in each exercise.

Patients with aphasia demonstrate reduced vocabulary, e.g. they have difficulty naming things and expressing ideas. Therefore, illustrations of useful items have been included to provide stimuli for increasing vocabulary recall. The illustrations have been organized into categories, e.g. "Grooming," "Clothing," "Food," "Drinks," "Furniture," etc. so as to promote maximum recall of words within the same category.

The recommended procedure for using the illustrations in this section is as follows:

1. Show each picture to the patient as you name it. Have the patient repeat the name after you. If he is unable to repeat the word, break down the word into single sounds. Have him repeat each phoneme and then try to combine the sounds to form whole word.

2. When the patient is able to repeat the names of most pictures, he can proceed to the task of naming a picture on his own. Help the patient by giving him a clue to the name of the picture by supplying him with the initial sound of the word, e.g. make a hard "k" sound when presenting the picture of "coffee."

3. Often supplying a commonly used lead-in phrase, e.g. "A cup of _____," while presenting a picture of "coffee" is helpful in eliciting the correct response.

4. After the patient can name pictures of common objects with the help of initial sound cues and partial phrases, begin to reduce these cues and encourage the patient to name the illustrations without assistance.

5. For more advanced patients, the pictures provide an opportunity for structured conversational speech practice. Have the patient look at the illustrations and make a sentence using the key words depicted.

In addition to reduced vocabulary, many aphasic patients exhibit errors of grammar and syntax. Errors of grammar include improper usage of parts of speech such as nouns, pronouns, verbs, and prepositions and articles. For example, many patients confuse the use of pronouns "he" and "she." Exercises to stimulate correct usage of specific parts of speech have been included. Errors of syntax mean improper arrangement or word order. When writing and speaking some patients have a tendency to invert word order. Exercises to improve syntax have been provided. The patient is asked to arrange the words in the proper order so that the sentence makes sense; e.g. "Football watch I on TV to like." Corrected, it should read "I like to watch football on TV."

Furthermore, there are exercises to stimulate sentence formulation, e.g. a patient is given two key words, "read" and "book," and is told to construct a sentence, e.g. "I read a book." Lastly, there are paragraphs to be filled in with appropriate words. Practicing naming pictures, as well as correct grammar usage and syntax, enhances the recovery of all expressive language skills.

SAY THE OPPOSITE:

Directions: Read the word aloud, then have the patient supply the opposite. For example: if I say "hot," you say "cold."

hot _____

up _____

in _____

on _____

open _____

wet _____

good _____

true _____

left _____

rich _____

clean _____

sweet   _____

hello   _____

black   _____

empty   _____

early   _____

narrow   _____

shiny   _____

yes   _____

narrow   _____

difficult _____

far   _____

fast   _____

crooked   _____

man   _____

fancy   _____

SAY THE OPPOSITE:

Directions: Read the word aloud, then have the patient supply the opposite. For example: if I say "hot," you say "cold."

wrong _____

fat   _____

young _____

big   _____

tall   _____

heavy _____

quiet _____

ugly   _____

tight _____

easy   _____

start _____

near _____

top _____

loud _____

come _____

buy _____

ceiling _____

hard _____

new _____

ahead _____

slowly _____

honest _____

more _____

agree _____

expensive_____

OPPOSITES

Directions: The clinician reads these sentences aloud and the patient supplies the appropriate OPPOSITE word.

Example: **Ice is cold; soup is ___hot___ .**

A scream is loud; a whisper is _____.

Sugar is sweet; lemon is _____.

Mountains are high; valleys are _____.

Red light says stop; green light says _____.

You get up in the morning; you sleep at _____.

John is a boy; Mary is a _____.

Turn the light on; turn the light _____.

The window is closed; the window is _____.

Entrance means in; exit means _____.

A pillow is soft; a rock is _____.

Rhinestones are cheap; diamonds are _____.

This clock is slow; that clock is _____.

This dress costs more; that dress costs _____.

Those men are honest; this one is _____.

An elephant is heavy; a feather is _____.

THINGS THAT GO TOGETHER

Directions: Fill in a word that goes together with the word in the first column.

Example:

Bread and <u>butter</u>

hat _____

shirt _____

bacon _____

scotch _____

donuts _____

nurse _____

paper _____

cream _____

table _____

meat _____

robe _____

Stamp and _____

comb _____

pencil _____

pants _____

vinegar _____

sheets _____

necklace _____

eyes _____

buttons _____

sunny _____

ice _____

bat _____

THINGS THAT GO TOGETHER

Directions: Fill in a word that goes together with the word
in the first column.

Example: **Knife and** <u>fork</u>

mother _____

dessert _____

sister _____

husband _____

lettuce _____

pepper _____

needle _____

soap _____

shoes _____

salt _____

skirt _____

Cheese and _____

tea _____

cup _____

son _____

stocks _____

windows _____

pots _____

hammer _____

mop _____

washer _____

pad _____

nickels _____

WORD PAIRS

Directions: Supply the appropriate word to complete these common word pairs.

Example: **Radio and** _____TV_____

Apples and _____

Soup and _____

Ham and _____

Hands and _____

Man and _____

Arms and _____

Coffee and _____

Corn and _____

Black and _____

Lemons and _____

Soap and _____

Scotch and   _____

Door and   _____

Stocks and   _____

Syrup and   _____

Frankfurters and   _____

Soup and   _____

Bra and   _____

Peanut butter and   _____

Chocolate and   _____

Gold and   _____

Damp and   _____

Safe and   _____

SENTENCE COMPLETION

Directions: Complete these well-known proverbs with the
              appropriate missing word.

Example: **No news is good __news__ .**

Time waits for no _____.

Time heals all _____.

Look before you _____.

**A dog is a man's best
_____.**

**Make hay while the sun
_____.**

Haste makes _____.

**Money is the root of all
_____.**

Better late than _____.

**The early bird catches the
_____.**

Honesty is the best _____.

Fools rush in where angels fear to _____.

Penny wise and pound _____.

A penny saved is a penny _____.

SENTENCE COMPLETION

Directions: Complete these well-known proverbs with the appropriate missing word.

Example: **You can't see the forest for the ___trees___ .**

An apple a day keeps the doctor _____ .

Don't put all your eggs in one _____ .

Too many cooks spoil the _____ .

Two heads are better than _____ .

There's no place like _____ .

Don't count your chickens before they're _____ .

Don't cry over spilt _____ .

Nothing succeeds like _____ .

Practice makes _____.

You can't get blood out of a _____.

A cold hand, a warm _____.

Good news travels _____.

Nothing ventured, nothing _____.

ANSWERING "YES" AND "NO"

Directions: Ask these questions of the patient. Have him answer by saying "yes" and "no." (Proper lip position for starting these words is as follows: smiling for "yes," rounded for "no" with tongue tip raised.)

Say: Yes or No

Example: **Is your name Jack?**

Is your name Bob?

(Use patient's real name)

Are you at home?

Are you at the office?

Are you sleeping?

Are you awake?

Are you a man?

Are you a woman?

Is the light on?

Is the light off?

Is it daytime?

Is it nighttime?

Are you in bed?

Are you in a chair?

Are you in the hospital?

COMPLETE THESE PHRASES

Example: **A dozen** _eggs_

A stick of chewing _____

A gallon of unleaded _____

A pint of ice _____

A tube of tooth _____

A keg of _____

A glass of cold _____

A carton of _____

A roomful of _____

A pocketful of _____

A cup of black _____

A slice of roast _____

An acre of _____

A closet full of _____

COMPLETE THESE PHRASES

Example: **A bowl of _soup_**

A piece of apple _____

A cup of hot _____

A head of _____

A pot of fresh _____

A dish of vanilla _____

A drink of _____

A scrambled _____

A box of chocolate _____

A jar of grape _____

A dozen red _____

A loaf of white _____

A pinch of _____

A pair of sharp _____

SENTENCE COMPLETION

Directions:　Fill in these common phrases with the appropriate word.

Example:　**How are __you__ ?**

Fine, thank _____.

Pardon _____.

Let's go _____.

Come over _____.

Please sit _____.

Hurry _____.

Good _____.

See you _____.

Have a nice _____.

So long, good- _____.

What's _____?

FILL-IN SENTENCES

Directions: Finish these sentences with an appropriate word.

Example: **I want a cup of ___tea___ .**

I want a glass of orange _____.

I want a bowl of _____.

I want a slice of _____.

I want a piece of _____.

I want a dish of _____.

I want a bottle of _____.

I want a box of _____.

I want a loaf of _____.

I want a jar of _____.

I want a bunch of _____.

I want a pack of _____.

FILL-IN SENTENCES

Directions: Finish these sentences with an appropriate word.

Example: I put water in a ___glass___.

I put sugar in my _____.

I put beer in a _____.

I put tea in a _____.

I put butter on _____.

I put cheese on _____.

I put meat on a _____.

I put jam on _____.

I put milk in a _____.

I put cereal in a _____.

I put syrup on _____.

I put money in the _____.

I put clothes on a _____.

I put change in my _____.

I put lemon in my _____.

SENTENCE COMPLETION

Directions: Fill in the missing appropriate words. The clinician starts the sentence and the patient completes the thought. Any word that makes sense is acceptable.

Example: **Open the ___door___ .**

Blow your _____.

Wash your _____.

Answer the _____.

Shave your _____.

Wipe your _____.

Dial the _____.

Turn on the _____.

Call the _____.

Mail the _____.

Scrub my _____.

Brush your _____.

SENTENCE COMPLETION

Directions: Fill in missing appropriate words. The clinician starts the sentence and the patient completes the thought. Any word that makes sense is acceptable.

Example: **Close the <u>window</u> .**

Drive the _____ .

Sit in a _____ .

Sleep on a _____ .

Eat your _____ .

Comb your _____ .

Read the _____ .

Go to the _____ .

Write with a _____ .

Shave with a _____ .

Watch the _____ .

Put on your _____ .

SENTENCE COMPLETION

Directions: Fill in the missing word. The clinician says the beginning of the sentence and the patient completes the thought. Any word that makes sense is acceptable.

Example: **Coffee is made in a __pot__ .**

Toast is made in a _____.

Eggs are fried in a _____.

Cake is baked in the _____.

Salad is mixed in a _____.

Soup is served in a _____.

Ice cream is served in a _____.

Soda is served in a _____.

Steak is broiled on the _____.

Cereal is served in a _____.

SENTENCE COMPLETION

Directions: Fill in the missing appropriate words. The clinician starts the sentence and the patient completes the thought. Any word that makes sense is acceptable.

Example: **I shave with a_razor_ .**

I cut meat with a _____ .

I write with a _____ .

I wash with soap and _____ .

I dry myself with a _____ .

I wipe my nose with a _____ .

I eat with a knife and _____ .

I listen with my _____ .

I see with my _____ .

I clap with my _____ .

I stir coffee with a _____ .

I open the door with a _____ .

I wear shoes on my _____ .

COMPLETE THESE SENTENCES

Directions: Fill in the missing appropriate words. The clinician starts the sentence and the patient completes the thought.

Example: I write with a _pencil_ .

I lock the _____.

I drive a _____.

I ride the _____.

I drink from a _____.

I eat with a _____.

I wear a _____.

I press my _____.

I spend my _____.

I shave with a _____.

I drink a glass of _____.

I sleep in a _____.

COMPLETE THESE SENTENCES

Directions: Fill in the missing appropriate words. The clinician starts the sentence and the patient completes the thought.

Example: **I comb my   hair .**

I cook on the _____.

I like to watch _____.

I sit in a _____.

I like to play _____.

I sign my _____.

I listen to the _____.

I mail a _____.

I sew my _____.

I polish my _____.

I shampoo my _____.

I shave my _____.

COMPLETE THESE SENTENCES

Directions: Fill in the missing appropriate words. The clinician starts the sentence and the patient completes the thought. Any word that makes sense is acceptable.

Example: **I eat bread and butter .**

I drink a glass of _____.

I take my pills with _____.

I wear a wrist _____.

I like to watch _____.

I am sitting in a _____.

I go to sleep when I am _____.

I wear shoes and _____.

I drink a cup of _____.

My wife's name is _____.

My name is _____.

My doctor's name is _____.

FINISH THESE SENTENCES

Directions: Fill in the missing appropriate words. The clinician starts the sentence and the patient completes the thought. Any word that makes sense is acceptable.

Example: **I look out the <u>window</u>.**

I go for a _____.

I put on my _____.

I comb my _____.

I wash my _____.

I mail a _____.

I listen to the _____.

I shop at the _____.

I dial your _____.

I eat my _____.

I lock the _____.

FILL-IN SENTENCES

Directions: The clinician starts the sentence and the patient completes the thought. Any word that makes sense is acceptable.

Example: I am very___tired___.

I need a _____.

I like to go _____.

I feel very _____.

I drink some cold _____.

I eat a soft-boiled _____.

I watch the _____.

I went to the _____.

I use a comb and _____.

I have a pain in my _____.

I take a ride in a _____.

I call for _____.

I go to the _____.

I want to get _____.

I have an appointment with the _____.

I knock on the _____.

I rest my head on a _____.

I cover myself with a _____.

I close my eyes and go to _____.

People buy stocks and _____.

I go for a ride in a _____.

COMPLETE THESE SENTENCES

Example: I eat bacon and __eggs__ .

I take my pills with _____.

I eat lettuce and _____.

I wear a wrist-_____.

I like to go _____.

I take pictures with a _____.

I sent a letter to my _____.

I am getting _____.

I want to go _____.

I like to sit outside on the _____.

I am drinking a cup of _____.

I don't like a bath, I take a _____.

I use a comb and a _____.

I drink a glass of iced _____.

I wear a long-sleeved _____.

I need to take a _____.

He bought a new pair of _____.

I change the _____.

I drink coffee from a _____.

She must go on a _____.

I weigh myself on a _____.

My address is _____.

My phone number is _____.

FINISH THESE SENTENCES

Example: I eat bread and __butter__ .

I wear shoes and _____ .

I wash with soap and _____ .

I eat lettuce and _____ .

I eat a bagel and _____ .

I have cake and _____ .

I use a pen and _____ .

I use a knife and _____ .

I have a brother and a _____ .

I eat mashed potatoes and _____ .

I eat crackers and _____ .

I eat ice cream and _____ .

I eat cookies and _____ .

FINISH THESE SENTENCES

Example: I like apple __pie__ .

I drink a glass of _____.

I drink a cup of _____.

I eat bacon and _____.

I eat meat and _____.

I eat french fried _____.

I read the daily _____.

I wear eye-_____.

I wear a shirt and _____.

I eat a piece of _____.

I eat a bowl of _____.

I ride in a _____.

I want to go _____.

I feel _____.

SENTENCE COMPLETION

Directions: The clinician reads the beginning of the sentence; the patient is to supply the correct missing word.

Example: I read the newspaper or a __book__ .

I ride in a bus or a _____.

I drink coffee or _____.

I tell time by the clock or my _____.

I watch the sports and the _____.

I cut with scissors or a _____.

I listen to records or the _____.

I wash with soap and _____.

I eat with a knife and _____.

I wear shoes and _____.

I eat apples and _____.

I wear a jacket and a _____.

It looks like it's going to _____.

I hope you have a nice _____.

You are looking very _____.

The sun is _____.

The sky is _____.

FILL-IN SENTENCES

Directions: Complete these sentences with the appropriate word.

Example: I like to watch ___TV___.

Turn on the hot and cold
_____.

Don't forget to lock the
_____.

Please wipe my eye _____.

She is wearing a hat and a
_____.

I need a comb and a _____.

When it rains, you carry an
_____.

If it's too hot, you should
open the _____.

I sit on a couch or a _____.

I write with a pen or a
_____.

FILL-IN SENTENCES

Directions: Complete these sentences with the appropriate word.

Example: **You take a picture with a camera .**

You sit in a _____.

A man wears shoes and _____.

A woman carries a _____.

A man wears a shirt and a _____.

You wear a robe and _____.

He is wearing a sport _____.

I have to wind my _____.

I'd like a cup of _____.

I like to listen to the _____.

FILL-IN SENTENCES USING THESE PHRASES

Example:　On the wall, there is a <u>picture</u>.

On the floor, there is _____.

On the table, there is _____.

On the sink, there is _____.

On the ceiling, there is _____.

On the bed, there is _____.

On the desk, there is _____.

On the dresser, there is _____.

On the end table, there is _____.

On the shelf, there is _____.

On the stove, there is _____.

On the door, there is _____.

On the belt, there is a _____.

On the telephone dial, there are _____.

FILL-IN SENTENCES USING THESE PHRASES

Example: In my pocket, there is <u>money</u>.

In the bathroom, there is a _____.

In the bedroom, there is a _____.

In the kitchen, there is a _____.

In the closet, there are _____.

In the bakery, there are _____.

In the library, there are _____.

In the post office, there are _____.

In the pharmacy, there are _____.

In the hospital, there are _____.

In the bus, there are _____.

ANSWER THESE QUESTIONS

Example: **What do you put in your coffee?**   <u>cream</u>

What do you put in a safe?   _____

What do you put in a desk drawer?   _____

What do you put in a wallet?   _____

What do you put in your tea?   _____

What do you put in a salad?   _____

What do you carry in your pocket?   _____

What do you put on toast?   _____

What do you hang in the closet?   _____

**What do you put in
the bank?**   _____

**What do you put in
your cereal?**   _____

**What do you put in
the garage?**   _____

**What do you put on
pancakes?**   _____

**What do you put on
a birthday cake?**   _____

**What do you put in
the refrigerator?**   _____

**What do you put on
a frankfurter?**   _____

**What do you put on
an envelope?**   _____

ANSWER THESE QUESTIONS

Example: **What do we smoke?**

cigarettes

**What do we write
with?**   _____

**What do we kick
with?**   _____

**What do we cut
meat with?**   _____

What do we read?   _____

**What do we pour
water from?**   _____

**What do we cook
food on?**   _____

**What do we switch
on when it's dark?**   _____

**What do we use for
unlocking the door?**   _____

**What do we use for
sweeping the floor?**   _____

What do we use to
cover the floor? _____

What do we use for
playing golf? _____

What do we use for
playing tennis? _____

What vehicle do
you drive? _____

What do you put on
a letter for mailing? _____

What do you use to
find out how much
you weigh? _____

Where do you go if
you have a tooth-
ache? _____

Who do you call
if your pipes or
drains are out of
order? _____

Who do you call if
you are sick? _____

What do you use to
take pictures? _____

What do you tell
time with? _____

What do you write
with? _____

What do you use to
tell the date? _____

What do you use to
take your temper-
ature? _____

What do you spend? _____

What do you use
for shaving? _____

What do you dial? _____

What do you use
for sewing? _____

What do you use
to measure inches? _____

Where do you keep
medicines? _____

Where do you keep
ice cream? _____

Where do you find
a definition? _____

SYNONYMS

(Words That Have Similar Meaning)

Directions: Say a word that has a similar meaning.

Example: **talk**   _speak_

upset   _____

close by   _____

auto   _____

cheap   _____

spouse   _____

attorney   _____

prison   _____

home   _____

o.k.   _____

road   _____

NAMING SKILLS

ITEMS AROUND THE ROOM

Directions: The clinician points to items around the room and the patient tries to name the items.

table

chair

floor

ceiling

wall

television

couch

rug

radio

picture

This procedure is repeated for practicing naming body parts, clothing, items in the bedroom, bathroom, kitchen, etc.

NAMING SKILLS

Directions: The clinician uses the illustrations of useful objects in categories that are included in this section on the following pages. Pointing to the pictures, the patient is told to name the pictures by
saying "What is this?" If the patient is unable to
name the pictures, initial sound cues are given to
help elicit the correct response. For example:
using the illustrations of "Drinks" (page 195) a
hard "k" is spoken by the clinician to evoke the
word "coffee." In addition, a lead-in phase, such
as "I drink a cup of ____," is provided by the
clinician as a cue.

This procedure is repeated for all of the illustrations until the
patient can name the pictures without assistance.

GROOMING

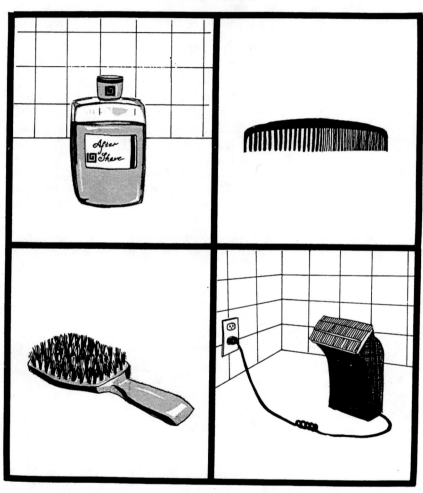

after shave lotion
brush

comb
electric razor

GROOMING

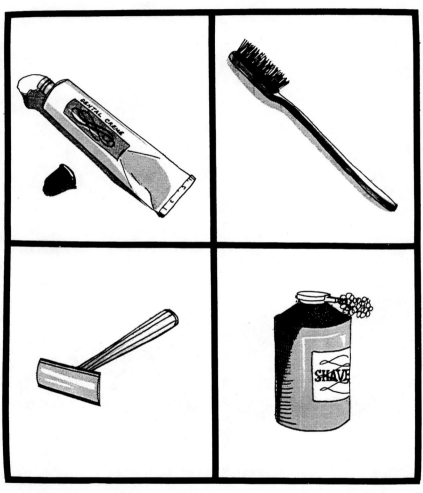

toothpaste   **toothbrush**
razor   **shaving cream**

GROOMING

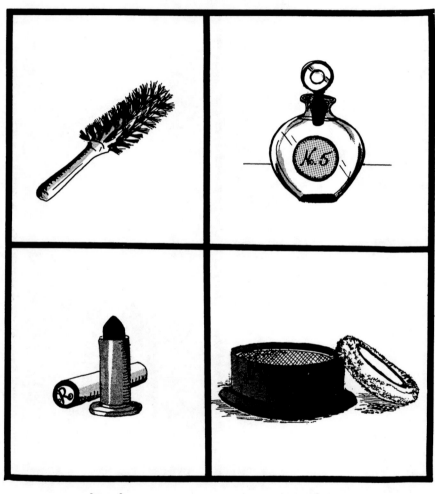

brush
lipstick

perfume
powder

GROOMING

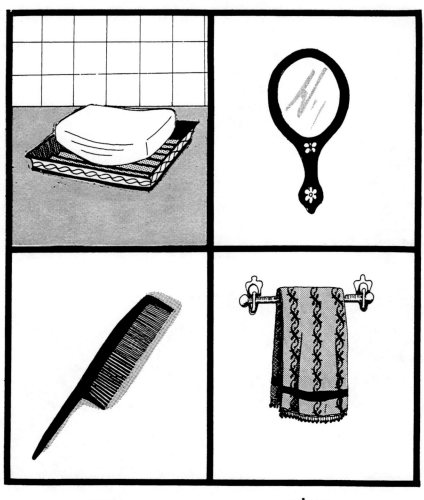

soap   mirror
comb   towel

CLOTHING

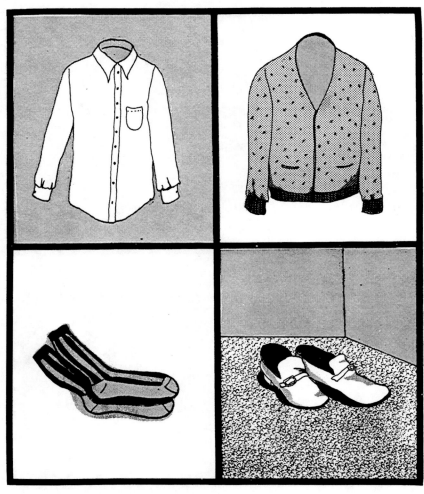

shirt   **sweater**
socks   **shoes**

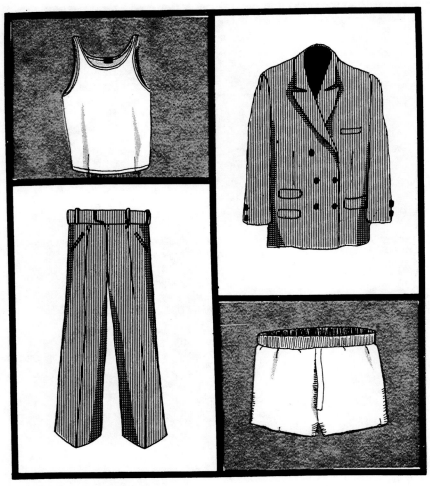

undershirt
pants

jacket
shorts

CLOTHING

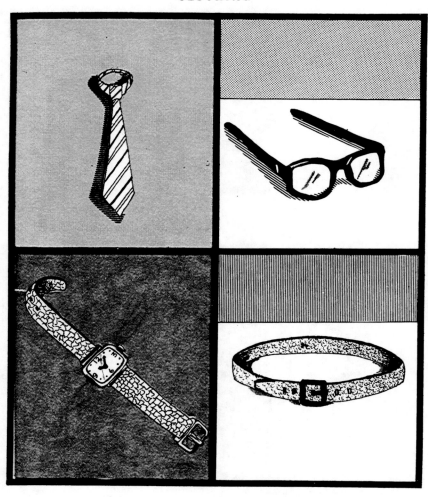

tie   **glasses**
watch   **belt**

CLOTHING

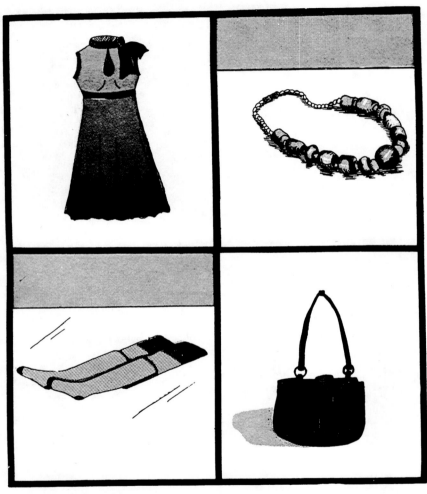

dress   **necklace**
stockings   **pocketbook**

CLOTHING

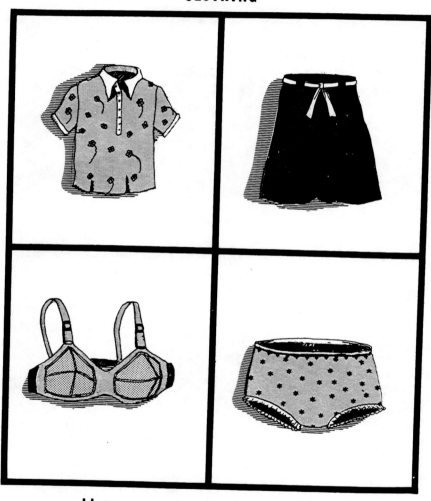

blouse
bra

skirt
underpants

FOOD

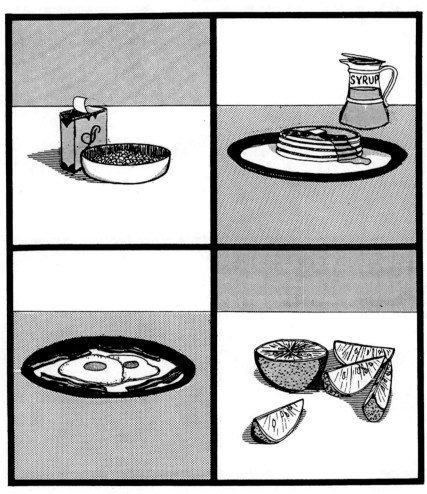

cereal
bacon and eggs

pancakes
oranges

FOOD

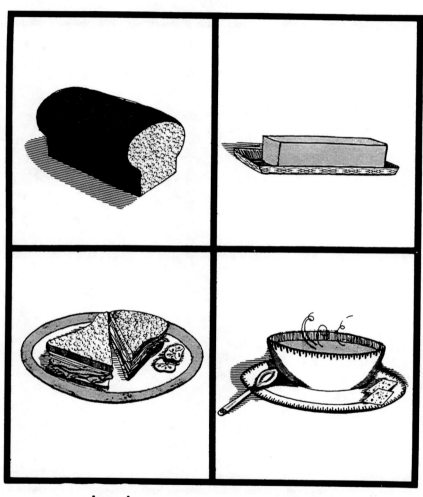

bread
sandwich

butter
bowl of soup

FOOD

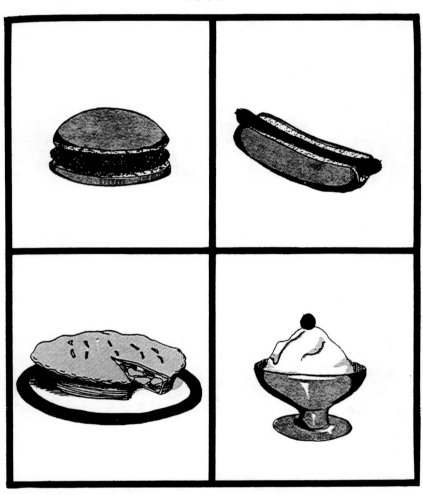

hamburger
pie

hot dog
ice cream

FOOD

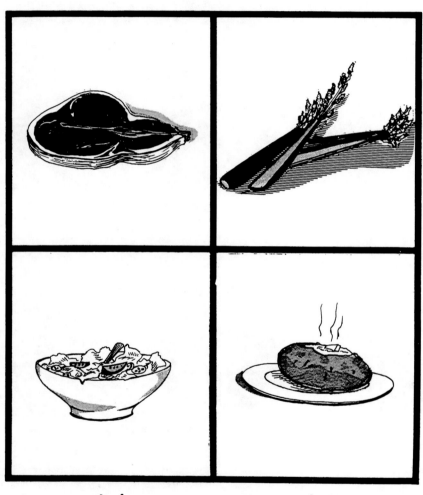

steak   celery
salad   potato

DRINKS

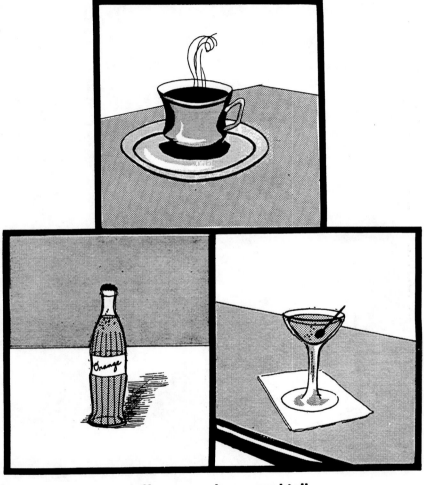

coffee   soda   cocktail

DRINKS

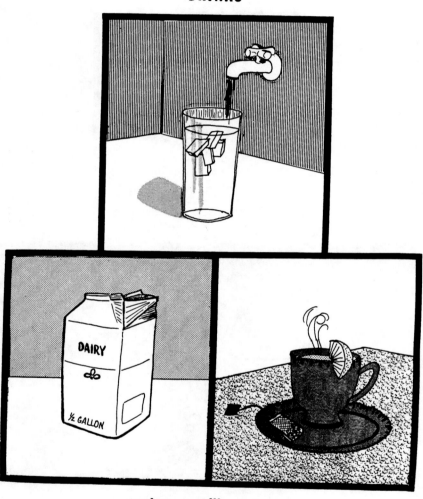

water   milk   tea

FURNITURE

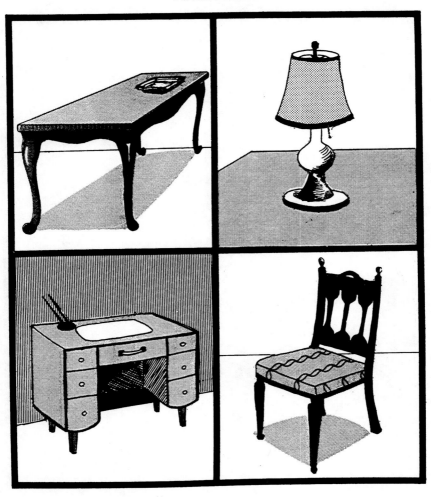

table
desk

lamp
chair

TABLEWARE

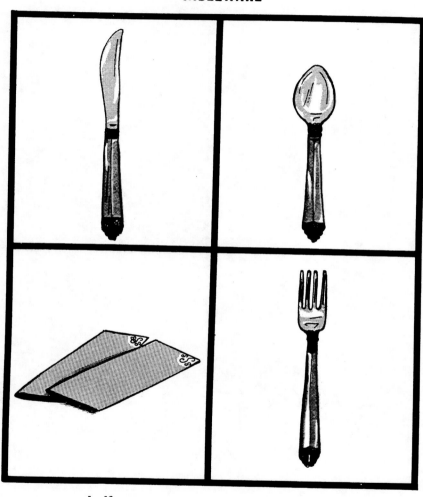

knife
napkin

spoon
fork

TABLEWARE

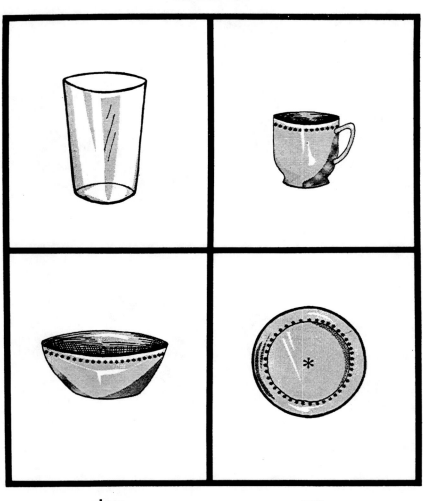

glass
bowl

cup
plate

TABLEWARE

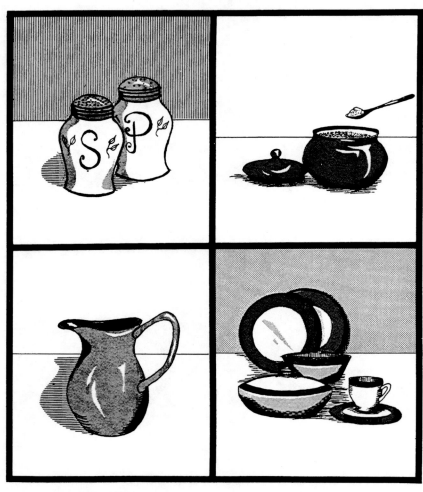

salt and pepper	**sugar**
pitcher	**dishes**

HOUSEHOLD ITEMS

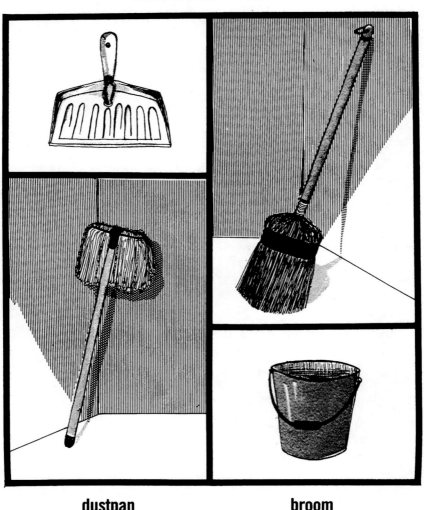

dustpan
mop

broom
pail

APPLIANCES

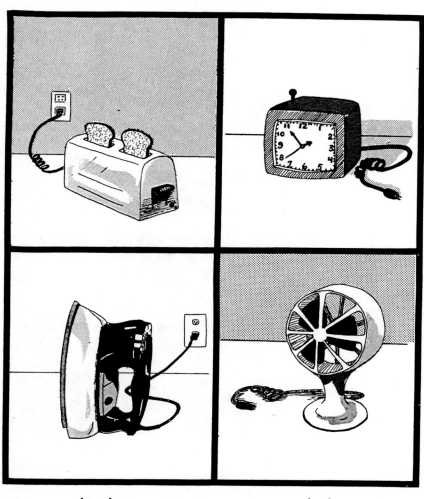

toaster
iron

clock
fan

APPLIANCES

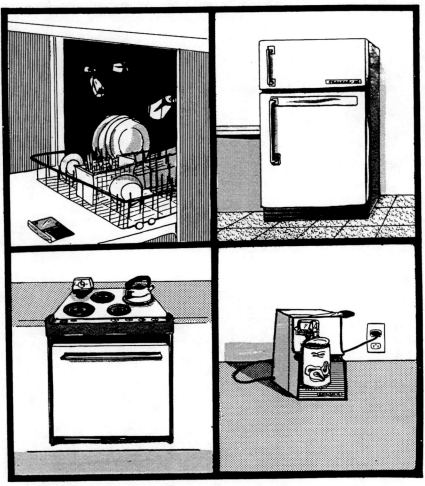

dishwasher
stove

refrigerator
can opener

ENTERTAINMENT

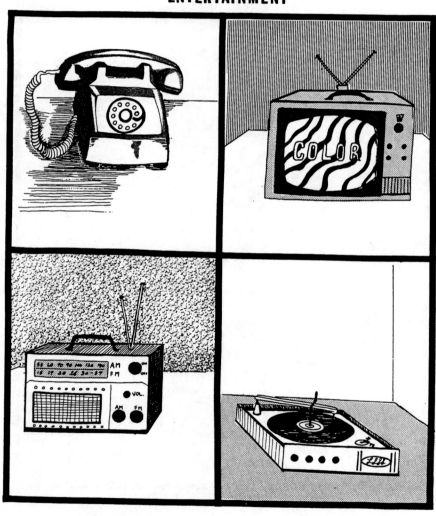

telephone
radio

television
record player

TRANSPORTATION

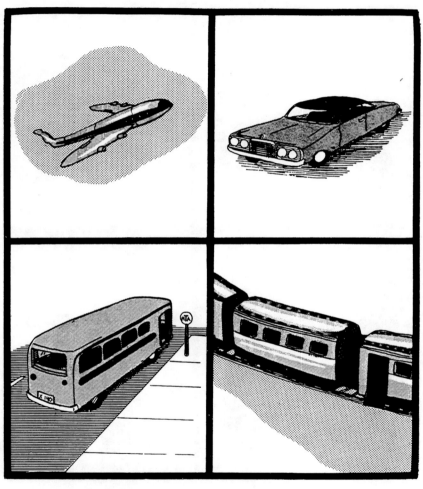

airplane
bus

car
train

UP AND DOWN

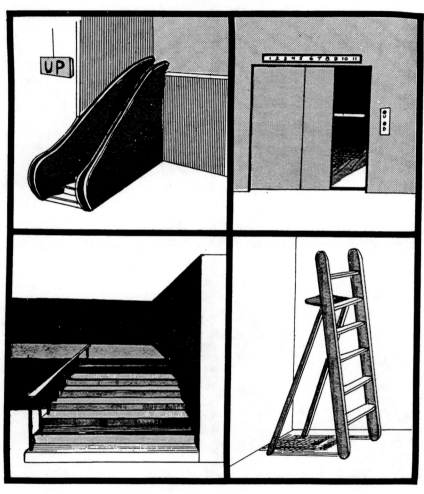

**escalator
stairs**

**elevator
ladder**

TOOLS

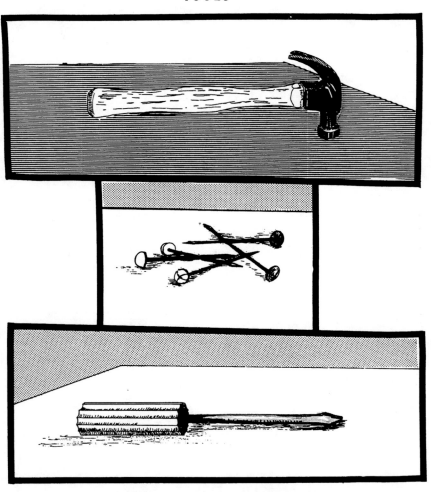

hammer   nails   screwdriver

GRAMMAR USAGE DRILL
VERBS

Directions: Tell what you do with these:

Example: **book**   _read_

eyeglasses _____

pen _____

knife _____

watch _____

ruler _____

key _____

hairbrush _____

razor _____

soap _____

handkerchief _____

GRAMMAR USAGE DRILL
VERBS

Directions: Tell what you do with these:

Example:	**feet**	**walk**
	eyes	_____
	ears	_____
	nose	_____
	chicken	_____
	eggs	_____
	airplane	_____
	dress	_____
	music	_____
	clock	_____
	phone	_____

GRAMMAR USAGE DRILL
VERBS

Directions: Tell what you can do with each of these items:

Example: **sink**	**wash**
hair	_____
stove	_____
TV	_____
chair	_____
telephone	_____
light	_____
door	_____
skirt	_____
shoes	_____
pills	_____
gum	_____
piano	_____
knife	_____

GRAMMAR USAGE DRILL

VERBS

Directions: Tell what you do with these:

Example:	**cigars**	smoke
	cereal	_____
	towels	_____
	magazine	_____
	letters	_____
	money	_____
	scissors	_____
	tissues	_____
	cup	_____
	eraser	_____
	sink	_____

GRAMMAR USAGE DRILL
VERBS

Directions: Tell what you can do with each of these items

Example: **pencil**	__write__
book	_____
car	_____
bus	_____
cup	_____
spoon	_____
letter	_____
clothes	_____
pen	_____
money	_____
razor	_____
water	_____
food	_____
bed	_____

GRAMMAR USAGE DRILL
VERBS

Directions: Tell what you do with these:

Example: **bread**   __eat__

towel   _____

knob   _____

television   _____

automobile   _____

blanket   _____

key   _____

bed   _____

scissors   _____

stove   _____

medicine   _____

clothes   _____

radio   _____

book   _____

GRAMMAR USAGE DRILL
VERBS

Directions: Tell what you do with BOTH these items:

Example: **Pen and pencil
are for**   <u>writing</u>

Soap and water   _____

Knife and fork   _____

Newspaper and books _____

Bus and car   _____

Shoes and socks   _____

Coffee and juice   _____

Clock and watch   _____

Apples and oranges   _____

Television and movies _____

Jacket and sweater   _____

Scissors and knife   _____

Radio and music   _____

GRAMMAR USAGE DRILL

Directions: Supply the missing verbs.

Example: **Read** the book.

_____ with eyeglasses.

_____ with a pencil.

_____ with a knife.

_____ time with a watch.

_____ with a key.

_____ with a razor.

_____ with a typewriter.

_____ with a hairbrush.

_____ with soap.

_____ with a handker-chief.

_____ from a cup.

GRAMMAR USAGE DRILL

Directions: Supply the missing verbs.

Example: I want to   <u>go</u>   to the bathroom.

I want to _____ the book.

I want to _____ my breakfast.

I want to _____ a new dress.

I want to _____ a letter to my friend.

I want to _____ to the doctor.

I want to _____ in the car.

I want to _____ better.

I want to _____ shopping.

I want to _____ my hair.

GRAMMAR USAGE DRILL

Directions: Supply the missing verbs.

Example: I want to __watch__ TV.

I want to _____ outside.

I want to _____ to sleep.

I want to _____ my din-
ner.

I want to _____ a nap.

I want to _____ the news-
paper.

I want to _____ on my
sweater.

I want to _____ my (son,
daughter) on the telephone.

I want to _____ a walk.

I want to _____ left alone.

GRAMMAR USAGE DRILL

Directions:　Supply the missing verbs.

Example:　I want to ___take___ a nap.

I need to _____ the doctor.

I need to _____ a vacation.

I have to _____ the broken lamp.

I have to _____ my exercises.

I have to _____ the beds.

I need to _____ my teeth.

I need to _____ a shave.

I have to _____ a telephone call.

I want to _____ my lunch.

GRAMMAR USAGE DRILL

Directions: Supply the missing verbs.

Example: **I have to __wash__ the dishes.**

I have to _____ the table.

I have to _____ the rent.

I have to _____ some new clothes.

I have to _____ my hair.

I have to _____ a shower.

I have to _____ my face and hands.

I need to _____ my medicine.

I need to _____ on a diet.

I need to _____ the letters.

GRAMMAR USAGE DRILL

Directions: Supply the missing verbs.

Example: I ___go___ to the store.

I _____ a sandwich.

I _____ money.

I _____ a sweater.

I _____ to the bathroom.

I _____ the doctor.

I _____ television.

I _____ the newspaper.

I _____ to music.

I _____ the checks.

GRAMMAR USAGE DRILL

Directions: Supply the missing verbs.

Example: I __wash__ my hair.

I _____ the door.

I _____ in my bed.

I _____ with a towel.

I _____ with scissors.

I _____ bread.

I _____ a cup of coffee.

I _____ cigarettes.

I _____ on the stove.

I _____ my medicine.

I _____ the knob.

I _____ money.

GRAMMAR USAGE DRILL

Directions: Supply the missing verbs.

Use the words: take—use—have

Example: I **take** a bath.

I _____ the phone.

I _____ soap.

I _____ a suit.

I _____ my lunch along.

I _____ my pills.

I _____ a cold.

I _____ eyeglasses.

I _____ a shower.

I _____ a comb.

I _____ a napkin.

I _____ my own tooth-brush.

GRAMMAR USAGE DRILL

Directions: Fill in the appropriate preposition.
Use the words: <u>to</u> — <u>for</u>

Example: **Give it ____to___ me.**

What is that _____?

A chair is _____sitting.

Introduce the man _____ me.

Show me how _____ do it.

Hold this _____ me.

Help me look _____ it.

I listen _____ the radio.

I must go _____ the bathroom.

GRAMMAR USAGE DRILL

Directions: Fill in appropriate prepositions.

Use the words: to — for

Example: **I went ____to____ the bank.**

I want to go _____ the movies.

I wear glasses _____ reading.

I have to go _____ the bathroom.

I paid _____ the ticket.

I went _____ a check-up.

I went _____ the doctor's.

I work _____ a living.

I bought a present _____ you.

I gave the money _____ the landlord.

GRAMMAR USAGE DRILL

Directions: Fill in appropriate prepositions.
Use the words: at — to — for

Example: **I look ___at___ my watch.**

I paid _____ the picture.

I look _____ myself.

I searched _____ the key.

Give it _____ her.

Come _____ my house.

Meet me _____ five o'clock.

Shop _____ the store.

Buy supplies _____ my office.

Meet me _____ noon.

GRAMMAR USAGE DRILL

Directions: Fill in appropriate prepositions.

Use the words: to — at

Example: I went _____ to _____ the store.

I went _____ Dr. Miller.

Meet me _____ Saks Fifth Avenue.

I went _____ the movies.

I saw him _____ the Food Fair.

Stop it, _____ once.

Come with us _____ the park.

Let's go _____ the shopping center.

Leave it _____ my house.

Deliver it _____ her.

Give the check _____ the landlord.

Listen _____ the radio.

GRAMMAR USAGE DRILL

Directions: Fill in appropriate prepositions.

Use the words: <u>to</u> — <u>at</u>

Example: **Look ___at___ TV.**

Give it _____ me.

Look _____ me.

Give the book _____ me.

Listen _____ me.

See you _____ 2:00 p.m.

We eat _____ noon.

Meet me _____ Lincoln Road.

I saw him _____ the office.

Look _____ your face.

Listen _____ the music.

GRAMMAR USAGE DRILL

Directions: Fill in appropriate prepositions.

use the words: to — on — at

Example: **I listen ____to____ the news.**

I look _____ TV.

I listen _____ you.

Put _____ the dress.

I go _____ the bathroom.

Shop _____ the store.

Turn _____ the movie.

I go _____ the bank.

Sleep _____ a bed.

They met _____ the dance.

I go _____ sleep.

I want _____ go home.

Turn _____ the air conditioner.

GRAMMAR USAGE DRILL

Directions: Fill in appropriate prepositions.

Use the words: <u>in</u> — <u>on</u> — <u>at</u>

Example: I am ____in____ a hurry.

The coffee is _____ the cup.

The lamp is _____ the table.

She is _____ home.

She is _____ a rush.

It is _____ the floor.

Stop it, _____ once.

Look _____ me.

Put it _____ the box.

He is always _____ time.

Put it _____ the table.

Turn _____ the TV.

Look _____ the mirror.

GRAMMAR USAGE DRILL

Directions: Fill in appropriate prepositions.

Use the words: <u>on</u> — <u>in</u>

Example: **The money is ___on___ the dresser.**

The phone is _____ the table.

The letter is _____ the drawer.

The keys are _____ the dashboard.

The soap is _____ the sink.

The pillow is _____ the bed.

The sheet is _____ the wash.

The tissues are _____ the box.

The mirror is _____ the door.

The watch is _____ my arm.

The socks are _____ the laundry.

The picture is _____ the wall.

My clothes are _____ the closet.

Soak your feet _____ the tub.

Pack your clothes _____ the suitcase.

Put the cup _____ the saucer.

Put the picture _____ the frame.

Put your shoes _____ your feet.

GRAMMAR USAGE DRILL

Directions: Fill in appropriate prepositions.

Use the words: <u>in</u> — <u>of</u>

Example: **I am thinking ____of____ you.**

Look _____ your wallet.

Put the money _____ your pocket.

She speaks highly _____ you.

It is made _____ glass.

A table is made _____ wood.

Throw the paper _____ the basket.

Put the letter _____ the mailbox.

Sit _____ that chair.

She is _____ a hurry.

What do you think _____ him?

GRAMMAR USAGE DRILL

Directions: Fill in appropriate prepositions.

Use the words: <u>of</u> — <u>in</u> — <u>on</u>

Example: Look ____**in**____ the mirror.

I heard _____ him.

Put the money _____ your pocket.

Put the stamp _____ the envelope.

Put the glasses _____ your pocket.

Put the shoes _____ your feet.

Sit down _____ this chair.

I came here _____ a car.

I saw him _____ the movies.

I'll pick you up _____ twenty minutes.

Put the package _____ the table.

I left my wallet _____ the dresser.

GRAMMAR USAGE DRILL

Directions: Fill in appropriate prepositions.

Use the words: <u>to</u> — <u>on</u>

Example: Give the book ___to___ me.

The pot is _____ the stove.

The doctor is _____ call.

The switch is _____ the wall.

I talk _____ my grandchildren.

Give the money _____ the landlord.

I talk _____ the doctor.

I listen _____ the program.

I put the bandage _____ my arm.

I talk _____ the phone.

I am going _____ vacation.

I listen _____ the sym-phony.

GRAMMAR USAGE DRILL

Directions: Fill in appropriate prepositions.

Use the words: <u>to</u> — <u>for</u>

Example: I went ____to____ the bank.

I want to go _____ the movies.

I wear glasses _____ reading.

I have to go _____ the bathroom.

I paid _____ the ticket.

I went _____ a check-up.

I went _____ the doctor's.

I work _____ a living.

I bought a present _____ you.

I gave the money _____ the landlord.

GRAMMAR USAGE DRILL

Directions: Fill in appropriate word.

Use the words: <u>the</u> — <u>your</u>

Example: Open ___the___ door.

Close _____ door.

Wash _____ face.

Comb _____ hair.

Brush _____ teeth.

Wash _____ hands.

Wind _____ watch.

Eat _____ dinner.

Shave _____ face.

Close _____ window.

Answer _____ telephone.

Read _____ newspaper.

Wipe _____ nose.

GRAMMAR USAGE DRILL

Directions: Fill in the correct word.

Use the words: the — a — some

Example: ___The___ boy is on time.

He has _____ new car.

He had _____ good excuse.

_____ house caught on fire.

I had _____ orange juice.

He walks _____ dog.

Give me _____ towel.

I need _____ money.

I read _____ newspaper.

I write _____ letter.

I want _____ time off.

I ate _____ sandwich.

Turn on _____ TV.

GRAMMAR USAGE DRILL

Directions: Fill in proper pronoun.

Use the words: <u>he</u> — <u>she</u>

Example: ___<u>He</u>___ is a nice man.

_____ is a sweet girl.

_____ is a nice lady.

_____ wants his lunch.

_____ makes   her   son's lunch.

_____ is combing her hair.

_____ wears a dress.

_____ lost her purse.

_____ needs her medicine.

_____ and she are married.

_____ lost his wallet.

_____ wears a coat and tie.

_____ buys her own clothes.

_____ used his own brush.

GRAMMAR USAGE DRILL

Directions: Fill in proper pronoun.

Use the words: <u>He</u> — <u>She</u>

Example: **The girl is angry. <u> She </u> is upset.**

The man is tall. _____ is handsome.

Bob is the boss. _____ works hard.

Jane is on her way home. _____ is late.

Jack drives very well. _____ has a new car.

Harry talks a lot about politics. _____ is a fine speaker.

Bill is very helpful. _____ is strong and healthy.

Helen is sixty-five. _____ doesn't look her age.

George is a lawyer. _____
is very successful.

Eleanor is pretty. _____
used to be a model.

GRAMMAR USAGE DRILL

Directions: Fill in the proper pronoun.

Use the words: his — her

Example: **Bob wants to eat ___his___ dinner.**

Jane was fired from _____ job.

Mary likes to entertain _____ friends.

Sally cleans _____ house.

Louise took _____ vacation in July.

Bob brought _____ lunch from home.

Marie plays golf with _____ friends.

George works with _____ father.

Sue plays cards with _____ sister.

He combs _____ hair.

She wears _____ clothes well.

Kathy packed _____ suit-case.

Rose ate _____ breakfast.

She has _____ hair done every Saturday.

GRAMMAR USAGE DRILL

Directions: Fill in appropriate pronoun.

Use the words: <u>you</u> — <u>me</u>

Example: How do __you__ do?

Thank _____ very much.

I'll see _____ later.

How nice to meet _____!

Where are _____ going?

What time are _____ coming back?

Give it to _____.

I will allow _____ to leave soon.

Leave _____ alone.

_____ had better hurry up.

Let _____ go now.

Give the book to _____.

_____ can do it yourself.

I will drive _____ in my car.

Let _____ have it.

Speak to _____ yourself.

GRAMMAR USAGE DRILL

Directions: Fill in the blank to complete the sentence.

Use the words: a — the — my

Example: **I take _____a_____ bath.**

I take _____ trip.

I take _____ chance.

I take _____ ride.

I take _____ time.

I take _____ temperature.

I take _____ vitamins.

GRAMMAR USAGE DRILL

Directions:　Fill in the blank to complete the sentence.

Use the words:　a — the

Example:　I take ____a____ walk.

I take _____ swim.

I take _____ nap.

I take _____ vacation.

I take _____ medicine.

I take _____ drink.

I take _____ lesson.

I take _____ taxi.

I take _____ test.

I take _____ shower.

GRAMMAR USAGE DRILL

Directions:　Fill in the blank to complete the sentence.

Use the words:　a — the — his

Example:　**He talks on ___the___ phone.**

He takes _____ walk.

He drinks _____ cup of coffee.

He puts on _____ shirt.

He closes _____ eyes.

He mails _____ letters.

He reads _____ paper.

He goes to _____ doctor.

He goes to _____ bank.

He signs _____ check.

He washes _____ face.

GRAMMAR USAGE DRILL

Directions: Fill in the blank to complete the sentence.

Use the words: a — the — her

Example: **She combs ___her___ hair.**

She takes _____ vacation.

She washes _____ hands.

She looks in _____ mirror.

She opens _____ door.

She brushes _____ teeth.

She looks at _____ menu.

She eats _____ dinner.

She buys _____ ticket.

She watches _____ TV.

She turns on _____ light.

GRAMMAR USAGE DRILL

Directions: Fill in the correct verb, so as to agree with the subject.

Example:

**I walk my dog.
He __walks__ his dog.**

**I dry my hands.
He _____ his hands.**

**I take my medicine.
He _____ his medicine.**

**I need some money.
He _____ some money.**

**I wind my watch.
He _____ his watch.**

**I drink my coffee.
He _____ his coffee.**

**I brush my teeth.
He _____ his teeth.**

**I use a towel.
She _____ a towel.**

I comb my hair.
She _____ her hair.

I write a letter.
She _____ a letter.

I sign a check.
She _____ a check.

I read the paper.
She _____ the paper.

I make the bed.
She _____ the bed.

I wash the dishes.
She _____ the dishes.

I cut the paper.
She _____ the paper.

GRAMMAR USAGE DRILL

Directions: Fill in the correct past tense of the verb.

Example: I walk my dog.
Yesterday I <u>walked</u> my dog.

I wash my face.
Yesterday I _____ my face.

I climb the stairs.
Yesterday I _____ the stairs.

I drive a car.
Yesterday I _____ my car.

I take my pills.
Yesterday I _____ my pills.

I talk on the phone.
Yesterday I _____ on the phone.

I go to the store.
Yesterday I _____ to the store.

I write with a pencil.
Yesterday I _____ with a pencil.

I need a loan.
Yesterday I _____ a loan.

I carry the packages.
Yesterday I _____ the packages.

I try my best.
Yesterday I _____ my best.

I am hungry.
Yesterday I _____ hungry.

I wish for something.
Yesterday I _____ for something.

I thank the man.
Yesterday I _____ the man.

I turn the knob.
Yesterday I _____ the knob.

GRAMMAR USAGE DRILL

Directions: Supply the correct plurals.

Example: **This is a shoe.
Those are a pair of __shoes.__**

**This is a dress.
Those are _____.**

**This is a phone.
Those are _____.**

**This is a house.
Those are _____.**

**This is a book.
Those are _____.**

**This is a chair.
Those are _____.**

**This is a child.
Those are _____.**

**This is a boy.
Those are _____.**

**This is a girl.
Those are _____.**

This is a man.
Those are _____.

This is a mouse.
Those are _____.

This is a foot.
Those are _____.

This is a tree.
Those are _____.

SENTENCE FORMULATION

Directions: Answer these questions using the preposition: at

Example: # Where do you buy meat?
I buy meat at the butcher.

Where do you buy clothes?
I buy clothes _____.

Where do you make a deposit?
I make a deposit _____.

Where do you play tennis?
I play tennis _____.

Where do you buy drugs?
I buy drugs _____.

Where do you buy gas?
I buy gas _____.

Where do you buy stamps?
I buy stamps _____.

Where do you buy shoes?
I buy shoes _____.

Where do you see a movie?
I see a movie _____.

Where do you get your teeth
fixed?
I get my teeth fixed _____.

Where do you get prescription glasses?
I get my prescription glasses
_____.

Where do you get a haircut?
I get a haircut _____.

Where do you get your dirty
clothes washed?
I get my clothes washed ____
_____.

SENTENCE FORMULATION

Directions: Answer these questions using the preposition: <u>on</u>

Example: **Where is the picture?**
The picture is <u>on the wall.</u>

Where is the clock?
The clock is _____.

Where is the doorbell?
The doorbell is _____.

Where is the mirror?
The mirror is _____.

Where is the rug?
The rug is _____.

Where is the phone?
The phone is _____.

Where is the pillow?
The pillow is _____.

Where is the blanket?
The blanket is _____.

Where is the ashtray?
The ashtray is _____.

Where is the lamp?
The lamp is _____.

Where is the book?
The book is _____.

SENTENCE FORMULATION

Directions: Answer these questions using the preposition: <u>on</u>

Example: # Where is the curtain?
The curtain is <u>on the window.</u>

Where is the light switch?
The light switch is ＿＿＿＿＿.

Where is your watch?
My watch is ＿＿＿＿＿＿.

Where is the light?
The light is ＿＿＿＿＿＿＿.

Where is your belt?
My belt is ＿＿＿＿＿＿＿.

Where is your ring?
My ring is ＿＿＿＿＿＿＿.

Where are your socks?
My socks are ＿＿＿＿＿＿.

Where are your shoes?
My shoes are ＿＿＿＿＿＿.

Where do you put your hat?
I put my hat _____.

Where do you put sheets?
I put sheets _____.

SENTENCE FORMULATION

Directions: Make a sentence by filling in the subject and verb.

Example: ____I____ __eat__ apples and oranges.

____ ____ bananas and pears.

____ ____ cake and cookies.

____ ____ milk and beer.

____ ____ coffee and tea.

____ ____ peas and carrots.

____ ____ water and juice.

____ ____ shirt and tie.

____ ____ shoes and socks.

____ ____ soap and water.

____ ____ ice cream and cake.

SENTENCE FORMULATION

Directions: Make a sentence by filling in the subject and verb.

Example: __I__ __eat__ bread and butter.

___ ___ with a knife and fork.

___ ___ a blouse and skirt.

___ ___ a hat and coat.

___ ___ in a sofa or a couch.

___ ___ with pots and pans.

___ ___ with a needle and thread.

___ ___ to the radio and to music.

___ ___ corn and beans.

___ ___ a magazine and newspaper.

___ ___ with a washcloth and sponge.

SENTENCE FORMULATION

Directions: Make a sentence by filling in the subject and verb.

Example: <u>I</u> <u>drink</u> coffee and juice.

____ ____ with a pen and pencil.

____ ____ in a taxi and bus.

____ ____ at the clock and watch.

____ ____ movies and TV.

____ ____ with a knife and scissors.

____ ____ a horn and whistle.

____ ____ with a tissue and handkerchief.

____ ____ sneakers and sandals.

____ ____ on the stove and oven.

____ ____ the flowers and plants.

SENTENCE FORMULATION

Directions: Make a sentence using these words:

Example: I <u>need</u> to <u>buy</u> some <u>bread.</u>

1.   need   buy   bread

2.   put   stamp   letter

3.   going   buy   present

4.   eat   breakfast   9:00 a.m.

5.   put   letter   mailbox

6.   need   glasses   reading

7.   have   go   bathroom

8.   put   money   bank

9.   want   go   movies

10.   need   wash   hair

11.   speak   friend   phone

12.   went   doctor   check-up

SENTENCE FORMULATION

Directions: Make a sentence using these words:

Example: I <u>read</u>   a   <u>book</u>

1.	read	book
2.	drawing	picture
3.	write	pencil
4.	talks	phone
5.	wash	soap
6.	watching	television
7.	listen	music
8.	ride	car
9.	look	mirror
10.	go	bathroom
11.	take	shower
12.	reads	paper

SENTENCE FORMULATION

Directions: Make a sentence using these words:

Example: I <u>write</u> with a <u>pen.</u>

1. write   pen

2. drink   coffee

3. mails   letter

4. get   haircut

5. goes   store

6. eat   breakfast

7. swimming   pool

8. make   deposit

9. signs   check

10. wearing   glasses

11. call   appointment

12. going   doctor

SENTENCE FORMULATION

Directions: Make a sentence using these words:

Example: I <u>eat</u> my <u>dinner.</u>

1. eat   dinner

2. watch   television

3. goes   bathroom

4. sleeps   bed

5. cut   knife

6. going   shopping

7. spend   money

8. go   doctor

9. call   friends

10. have   pain

11. buys   groceries

12. washes   dishes

SENTENCE FORMULATION

Directions: Make a sentence using these words:

Example: **I <u>live</u> in a <u>house.</u>**

1. live   house

2. drink   cup

3. standing   feet

4. sits   chair

5. go   bed

6. slices   tomato

7. wears   shirt

8. comb   hair

9. shaves   face

10. take   shower

11. went   cafeteria

12. dial   telephone

SYNTAX PRACTICE

Directions: Unscramble these sentences so they make sense.

1. sit a chair in I

2. TV on the turn

3. phone please the answer

4. door who's the at?

5. I can you help?

6. number your what phone is?

7. time what it is?

8. door please the open

9. the where bathroom is?

10. better hope get I I

11. rush into don't anything

12. time take think to it over

13. down sit please

14. you see later, good-bye

SYNTAX PRACTICE

Directions: Unscramble these sentences so they make sense.

1.   to go shopping I want

2.   football on TV I watch to like

3.   everyday shave I have to

4.   shampoo I my hair week once a

5.   make deposit I a at the bank

6.   called I the Social office Security

7.   going out I'm evening this

8.   be back I'll at o'clock 10

9.   me later call at home

10.   hungry, I'm want I to eat

11.   buy new car a I to want

12.   take my need I to medicine

Directions: Read aloud and fill in blanks with appropriate missing words. Then answer questions.

Getting Up

A woman has had a good night's sleep and now it is morning. She yawns and stretches and gets out of _____. She washes her _____. She brushes her _____. She combs her _____. She puts on her _____. She eats her _____. Now she is ready to go _____.

1. What time of day is it now?

2. What meal did she eat?

3. Name three things you do when you get up.

4. What do you usually eat for breakfast?

Directions: Read aloud and fill in blanks with appropriate missing words. Then answer questions.

Getting Dressed

A man wears a "T"- _____ and under _____. He wears shoes and _____. He wears a long-sleeved _____. He wears a pair of _____. He wears a wrist-_____. He puts on his eye-_____. On his finger, he wears a _____. When he gets dressed up, he wears a jacket and _____. Around his waist, he wears a _____. When it's cool, he wears a woolen _____.

1. What is the man doing?

2. What does he wear on his feet?

3. What does he wear around his waist?

4. What does he wear to keep him warm?

5. What are you wearing now?

ADVANCED FILL-IN SENTENCES

Directions: Read aloud and fill in blanks with appropriate missing words. Then answer questions.

<u>Grooming</u>

To wash, I use soap and _____. To brush my teeth, I use toothpaste and tooth-_____. A man shaves with a _____. He uses shaving _____. He uses after-shave ____. He dries off with a _____. He uses a comb and _____. Sometimes he uses an electric _____.

1. What is the man doing in the bathroom?

2. What do you use to shave yourself?

3. What do you use to wash yourself?

4. What do you do with a towel?

ADVANCED FILL-IN SENTENCES

Directions: Fill in appropriate words. Then answer questions.

Making Coffee

The man is _____ a pot of coffee.
He puts the coffee on the _____.
He waits for the water to _____.
When it boils, the coffee will be
_____. He _____ off the stove.
He _____ the coffee into the cup.
He puts the cup on a _____. To
make it sweet, he _____ some
_____ in the coffee. He _____
it with a spoon. He _____ a while
for it to cool. Now he is going to
_____ the coffee.

1. What is the man doing?

2. What does he cook on?

3. Where does he pour the coffee?

4. What does he add to the coffee?

5. What do you like in your coffee?

ADVANCED FILL-IN SENTENCES

Directions: Fill in missing appropriate words. Then answer questions.

Retiring for Bed

The woman is getting ready for bed. First, she takes a _____. Then, she brushes her _____ and washes her _____. She then puts on her night_____. Then she climbs into _____. She reads the _____ or watches _____. Then, she falls _____.

1. What time of day is it?

2. What do you do with you clothes before going to bed?

3. Do you prefer a bath or a shower?

4. Do you prefer reading or watching television?

ADVANCED FILL-IN SENTENCES

Directions: Fill in appropriate words. Then answer questions.

Buying Shoes

The man tries on a pair of _____.
He looks in the _____. He likes
the way the shoes _____. They
feel _____. He decides to buy the
_____. He pays for the _____.
He takes the shoes and goes _____.

1. What did the man buy?

2. What kind of store was he in?

3. How did the shoes fit?

4. What color shoes are you wearing?

5. What are they made of?

ADVANCED FILL-IN SENTENCES

Directions: Fill in appropriate words. Then answer questions.

Fixing the TV

The TV is not working properly. The _____ is blurred. The repairman comes to _____ the television. He changes the _____. The picture is improved. Now the TV has been _____. The customer pays the _____. The repairman leaves the _____.

1. What is wrong with the TV?

2. Who do you call to fix the TV?

3. Do you like to watch television?

4. In what room is your TV?

5. What is your favorite TV program?

ADVANCED FILL-IN SENTENCES

Directions: Fill in missing appropriate words. Then answer questions.

Preparing Dinner

First, the woman goes shopping. She goes in her _____ to the grocery _____. She takes a shopping _____ and buys all the _____. She _____ the groceries home. She unpacks the bags and puts the things in the _____. She sets the _____. She heats the food on the _____. When it's ready she serves the _____. After she has eaten dinner, she clears the _____. She washes the dirty _____. Then she sits down to _____.

1. Where did the woman buy the groceries?
2. What does she do with the groceries when she gets home?
3. What does she do after eating her dinner.
4. Tell what you ate for dinner last night.

ADVANCED FILL-IN SENTENCES

Directions: Fill in missing appropriate words. Then answer questions.

At the Doctor's Office

I got up early this _____. I didn't feel _____. I had a bad _____. I decided to call the _____. I made an _____ to see him. I went to his office by _____. He examined me and took my blood _____. He prescribed some _____. I must return to his _____ in one week.

1. Where did the man go?

2. How did he feel?

3. What did the doctor do?

4. What is your doctor's name?

ADVANCED FILL-IN SENTENCES

Directions: Fill in the appropriate words. Then answer questions.

At the Dentist

The patient is seated in the _____. The nurse puts the apron around his _____. The dentist looks into the patient's _____. He finds some _____. He drills the teeth and _____ the cavity. When the dentist is finished, the nurse removes the apron and the patient is ready to _____. The patient pays his _____ and makes another _____.

1. What kind of office is the man going to?

2. What does the dentist find?

3. What does the dentist do?

4. What is your dentist's name?

5. When was your last dental visit?

ADVANCED FILL-IN SENTENCES

Directions: Fill in appropriate words in blanks. Then answer questions.

At the Barber Shop

The man goes to the barber _____. He sits in the _____. The barber puts the apron around his _____. The customer tells him he wants a shave and a _____. The barber cuts his _____. The man looks in the _____ to see himself. The customer pays the _____ and leaves the _____.

1. Where is the man?

2. Who cuts his hair?

3. What else does he want done?

4. Who cuts your hair?

5. How much does it usually cost?

ADVANCED FILL-IN SENTENCES

Directions: Fill in missing appropriate words. Then answer questions.

At the Supermarket

A young lady is going _____. She takes a shopping _____. She goes up and down the _____. She goes to the meat department and selects a good piece of _____. She buys some bread, coffee, and _____. She takes her groceries to the _____. She puts them on the _____ and the cashier tells her how much she has to _____. She opens her _____ and pays the _____. The groceries are put in a _____. Then the bagboy helps carry the packages to her _____.

1. Where is she shopping?
2. What did she buy?
3. Who does she pay?
4. Where do you usually buy you groceries?
5. How much do you usually spend each week?

ADVANCED FILL-IN SENTENCES

Directions: Fill in appropriate words. Then answer questions.

At the Bank

A woman needs some money, so she _____ to her bank. She writes a _____ for $100. The teller instructs her to _____ the check and write her address and phone _____ on the back. The teller asks her how she would like the _____. She says she wants it in twenty dollar _____. The teller gives her _____ twenties. The woman says thank _____. After cashing the _____, she is ready to _____ the bank.

1. Where do you cash a check?

2. Where do you endorse the check?

3. What amount was the check?

4. How many bills did she receive?

5. What is the name of your bank?

ADVANCED FILL-IN SENTENCES

Directions: Fill in sentences with appropriate words. Then answer questions.

My Birthday

Today is my _____. I will be fifty _____ old. We are going to _____. My wife is making me a birthday _____. She has ordered a _____. She has invited many of my _____. She has given me a lovely _____. At the party we are serving cake and _____. My friends are due to _____ at 8 o'clock. This is a nice way to celebrate my _____.

1. What is the special occasion?

2. How old is the man?

3. Is he single or married?

4. What time is the party?

5. When is your birthday?

6. How did you celebrate it this year?

ADVANCED FILL-IN SENTENCES

Directions: Fill in appropriate words. Then answer questions.

Going to the Movies

A couple wants to see a movie. So they look up the time schedule in the _____. The husband _____ a comedy. The wife likes a mystery. They decide on a comedy. They _____ to the theater in their car. There is a long line for _____. The tickets cost $3.75 each. After they go inside and sit down they decide they want something to _____. They buy some _____ and a glass of _____. They both _____ the movie and laughed a lot.

1. Where did the couple go?
2. How did they find out the time schedule?
3. What kind of movie did they see?
4. How much did the tickets cost?
5. What did they eat at the movies?
6. What type of movie do you prefer?

ADVANCED FILL-IN SENTENCES

Directions: Fill in appropriate words. Then answer questions.

At the Drug Store

The man needs his prescription _____. He goes into the _____ store. He gives the prescription to the _____. He is told he will have to _____ fifteen minutes. He does some other shopping in the meantime. He buys some razor _____, some soap, and some shaving ____. He _____ back in fifteen minutes. Now his prescription is _____. He picks it _____ and asks _____ much he will have to _____. He pays the _____ and leaves the drug_____.

1. Where do you get a prescription filled?
2. How long did the man have to wait?
3. What other items did the man buy while waiting?
4. Where do you usually buy your drugs?

READING DEVELOPMENT SKILLS

A) Comprehension of written material

B) Oral reading of words and useful phrases, phonic drills, words that look similar

C) Money concepts

D) Time-telling practice with illustrated clocks

E) Advanced oral reading selection

READING DEVELOPMENT
SKILLS

IN ADDITION TO speech and language difficulties many aphasic patients have reading difficulties. Problems associated with reading can include difficulty in understanding written material and also in reading orally. These difficulties may appear separately or in combination.

It is essential that the patient understand what he is reading. Begin by teaching comprehension of simple written directions, e.g. "raise your hand," "close your eyes," etc.; have the patient read the directions silently and follow the written command. Exercises for this type of practice have been included. "Yes" and "no" questions, e.g. "Are you in the hospital?", *yes* or *no,* have also been included. The patient must read the question silently and point to the correct word to indicate comprehension of the written material.

Once it is learned that the patient understands what he is reading as demonstrated by his ability to follow written directions and point to correct answers to silent questions, he can then proceed to the exercises included to improve oral reading skills. First have the patient read in unison with the speech pathologist or family member. As he improves have him read aloud on his own. Improving oral reading skills has proven effective in recall of all expressive language skills, namely; speech, vocabulary, and writing.

The reading exercises progress in order of difficulty. First, there are word lists in which only the initial consonant differs, but the vowel sounds remain the same, for example: "Tie, Pie, Buy," etc. Next, there are lists of words that differ by one or two letters. Many patients have difficulty reading words that look similar, for example: "Buy — Boy" "Well — Will," and words that have letters transposed or reversed, e.g. "Dog — God." In addition, there are lists of words that sound the same but have different spellings and meanings, e.g. "Cent, Sent," "Blue, Blew."

Next, there are short sentences to be read aloud. These sentences begin with the same words but end differently, e.g. "I feel tired," "I feel sick," "I feel hungry," etc.

In addition, many aphasic patients demonstrate impaired ability to tell time and read numbers correctly aloud. Therefore, several clocks for time-telling practice have been included along with exercises specifically involving "o'clock," "half-past," "quarter of," and "quarter after." It is also recommended that a large-faced wristwatch or clock may be used for this practice.

Since many patients have difficulty with oral reading of numbers and doing simple math problems, exercises in addition, subtraction and money concepts have been included. It may be helpful to use actual coins and dollar bills when figuring money problems.

When the patient is able to read short sentences with minimal difficulty and to tell time fairly well, he should proceed to reading short paragraphs aloud. Questions on the contents of each paragraph are provided so that the patient's comprehension, retention, and ability to rephrase the contents can be tested.

Practicing retelling the main ideas helps in the language recall process that is necessary for recovery of conversational speech.

READING COMPREHENSION

Directions: Read this silently and follow these commands.

Raise your hand.

Open your mouth.

Shake your head "no".

Stick out your tongue.

Close your eyes.

Point to the ceiling.

Touch your nose.

Point to the door.

Make a fist.

Put your hand on your chest.

COMPREHENSION OF YES AND NO

Directions: Read these questions to yourself and put a check mark in the appropriate column.

Example: **Are all women short?**

	Yes	No
		√

1. **Are you a man?** _____ _____

2. **Are you a woman?** _____ _____

3. **Do you wear shoes on your feet?** _____ _____

4. **Do you speak Spanish?** _____ _____

5. **Are you tall?** _____ _____

6. **Have you eaten breakfast today?** _____ _____

7. **Do apples grow on trees?** _____ _____

8. **Does money grow on trees?** _____ _____

9. Does milk come
   from cows? _____ _____

10. Are there ten days
    in a week? _____ _____

11. Are there eleven
    months in a year? _____ _____

12. Are there sixty
    minutes in a hour? _____ _____

13. Are there stars
    in the sky? _____ _____

14. Do horses fly? _____ _____

15. Do all houses
    have fences? _____ _____

16. Do you wear
    warm clothes in
    hot weather? _____ _____

17. Do you put ice
    cream in the oven? _____ _____

READING COMPREHENSION

Directions: Read silently, then put a check mark in the appropriate column to indicate comprehension of the paragraph.

In Tarrytown, New York, a metal Indian which stood outside an estate was stolen. The article in the paper about the theft stated that "The Indian is 7 feet tall, weighs several hundred pounds, is brightly painted, dressed in battle garb, and is valued at $5,000." A reward for its recovery is posted.

	Yes	No
1. Was the Indian statue stolen?	____	____
2. Was the statue lightweight?	____	____
3. Was the statue taller than most men?	____	____

4. Was the statue
   brightly colored?   _____ _____

5. Did anyone find
   the stolen statue?   _____ _____

READING COMPREHENSION
WORD-PICTURE ASSOCIATIONS

Directions: Match words to pictures. Use the illustrations of useful items in categories provided in Section Three. Write down the names of the pictures on each page on a separate sheet of paper.

Example: # Clothing (p. 186)

shirt

sweater

shoes

socks

Show this list to the patient as he looks at the pictures. Have him match the words to the pictures by pointing to the word as you show him the picture. Repeat this procedure for each page of illustrations. Refer to pages 182 to 207.

ORAL READING

A B C D E F G H I J K

L M N O P Q R S T U V

W X Y Z

Directions: Match each letter below by pointing to the alphabet above, then say the letter aloud.

A	E	F	D	O
R	T	G	P	E
S	I	L	B	A
K	L	M	Q	U
W	Z	R	J	H
N	Y	V	X	C

ORAL READING

A B C D E F G H I J K

L M N O P Q R S T U V

W X Y Z

Directions: Use the alphabet above to help in reading orally and spelling individual letters of common abbreviations of trade names and stocks.

A.T.T.	I.B.M.	M.G.M.
G.E.	G.M.	R.C.A.
C.B.S.	N.B.C.	A.B.C.
S.C.M.	B.P.	I.T.T.
T.W.A.	U.A.L.	E.A.L.
U.S.S.	B.O.A.C.	A.&P.
M.D.	Ph.D.	D.D.S.
P.A.	LL.B.	Dr.

B.S.	**M.S.**	**M.A.**
Mr.	**Mrs.**	**Ms.**
A.F.L.	**C.I.O.**	**U.A.W.**
A.A.A.	**U.S.A.**	**U.S.S.R.**
U.N.	**N.Y.C.**	**L.A.**
N.J.	**S.C.**	**R.I.**

ORAL READING SKILLS

Directions: To assist in oral reading skills, have patient point to the letter in the words below, then to the same letter of the alphabet above while saying the letter aloud—then say the word aloud.

a b c d e f g h i j k

l m n o p q r s t u v

w x y z

he

she

me

bed

red

fed

bat

sat

fat

bell

well

tell

heat

seat

beat

call

ball

fall

wall

hall

take

make

bake

cake

lake

ORAL READING

Directions: Read aloud—words that rhyme.

sat	wet	start
pat	set	part
mat	jet	mart
hat	get	heart
chat	pet	chart
rat	met	art
flat	let	tart
that	bet	depart
spat	debt	cart
brat	net	dart
fat	regret	smart

ORAL READING

Directions: Read aloud—words that rhyme.

shoe	my	say
too	tie	day
few	pie	may
you	sigh	pay
new	try	they
view	guy	lay
cue	hi	way
blue	why	stay
two	by	pray
true	bye	ray
flu	buy	today
do	die	gay
due	high	delay
drew	fly	tray

ORAL READING

Directions: Read aloud—words that rhyme.

bed	cap	ear
head	map	hear
said	sap	dear
red	nap	clear
bread	wrap	tear
fed	strap	steer
shred	clap	queer
led	gap	mere
dread	rap	near
fled	tap	gear
Ted	trap	sheer
wed	snap	fear
instead	mishap	here
bled	lap	cheer

ORAL READING

Directions: Read aloud—words that rhyme.

air	no	me
hair	go	she
fair	so	be
stair	pro	fee
where	low	see
care	show	key
tear	know	tea
pear	dough	he
share	blow	three
square	toe	we
dare	row	ski
flair	bow	knee
scare	snow	tree
spare	slow	free

ORAL READING

Directions: Read aloud—words that look similar due to letter reversals and transpositions.

dim—mid

tea—eat

tug—gut

lap—pal

Ron—nor

trap—part

raw—war

pool—loop

on—no

dial—laid

but—tub

am—ma

meat—team

tease—seat

ORAL READING

Directions: Read aloud—words that look similar due to letter reversals and transpositions.

God—dog

pan—nap

leg—gel

lag—gal

saw—was

bed—deb

sag—gas

kitchen—chicken

pat—tap

tip—pit

not—ton

ten—net

bag—gab

leave—veal

knife—fine

ORAL READING

Directions: Read aloud—words that look similar.

mine mind	petal metal
sail tail	school stool
brink drink	cool tool
robe rope	damp stamp
rudder rubber	bread bead
try cry	locks socks
boils broils	watches watched

ORAL READING

Directions: Read aloud—words that look similar.

feel	caught
feet	taught
take	cough
talk	caught
wash	broke
was	brake
walk	dripped
wall	dropped
wilt	went
will	want
come	cold
comb	told
evening	warm
even	warn

ORAL READING

Directions: Read aloud—words that look similar.

ours **yours**	**his** **hers**
tire **tried**	**these** **theirs**
took **look**	**another** **other**
hair **here**	**better** **bitter**
above **about**	**combed** **climbed**
today **tonight**	**spilled** **slipped**
bar **par**	**will** **well**

ORAL READING

Directions: Read aloud—words that look similar.

nap **map**	**bush** **push**
radar **razor**	**hay** **day**
shaves **shades**	**fools** **tools**
wishing **fishing**	**rains** **raids**
wake **make**	**my** **pie**
we **me**	**bath** **path**
far **tar**	**east** **ease**

ORAL READING

Directions: Read aloud—words that sound alike but have different meanings.

sent **cent**	**bow** **beau**
hear **here**	**bee** **be**
hour **our**	**rain** **reign**
read **red**	**fare** **fair**
where **wear**	**see** **sea**
not **knot**	**boy** **buoy**
suite **sweet**	**blue** **blew**

ORAL READING

Directions: Read aloud—words that sound alike but have different meanings.

right	**pair**
write	**pear**
no	**toe**
know	**tow**
stair	**close**
stare	**clothes**
die	**buy**
dye	**bye**
read	**hair**
reed	**hare**
flee	**wrap**
flea	**rap**
wait	**maid**
weight	**made**

ORAL READING

Directions: Read aloud—useful phrases.

Hi there.

Come in.

Good-bye.

Thank you.

Pretty good

Good morning.

Good night.

Doctor, help me.

Nurse, come here.

So long.

No, thank you.

All right.

Pardon me.

Where have you been?

What did you say?

ORAL READING

Directions: Read these conversational phrases aloud—first in unison with the clinician, then on your own.

Hello.

How are you?

I feel fine.

What's new?

Nothing much.

Thank you.

Please.

Who's on the phone?

Hello, who's this?

Who's at the door?

Who's there?

ORAL READING

Directions: Read these conversational phrases aloud—first in unison with the clinician, then on your own.

Won't you come in?

Please sit down.

Do you want a drink?

Where's the bathroom?

It's over there.

I had a nice time.

What time is it?

I have to leave now.

Goodbye, see you soon.

Let's go.

ORAL READING

Directions: Read these conversational phrases aloud—first in unison with the clinician, then on your own.

OK.

That's right.

Excuse me.

Did you understand me?

What is your phone number?

Where are you going?

Of course.

Where have you been?

Please come again.

I am hungry.

Good afternoon.

You're welcome.

Did you have a good time?

Please help me.

What happened to her?

ORAL READING

Directions: Read these breakfast items aloud.

I want orange juice.

I want grapefruit.

I want prunes.

I want a bowl of cereal.

I want scrambled eggs.

I want boiled eggs.

I want poached eggs.

I want a piece of toast.

I want a roll.

I want a Danish.

I want a cup of coffee.

I want a cup of tea.

I want a glass of milk.

ORAL READING

Directions: Read these lunch items aloud.

I want a sandwich.

I want a bowl of soup.

I want a salad.

I want a hamburger.

I want a hot dog.

I want some eggs.

I want some bread.

I want a cup of coffee.

I want a cup of tea.

I want a glass of soda.

I want a glass of water.

I want Jell-O®.

I want cake.

I want some fruit.

ORAL READING

Directions: Read these dinner items aloud.

I want a glass of tomato juice.

I want a fruit cup.

I want a bowl of soup.

I want a salad.

I want a steak.

I want some chicken.

I want some fish.

I want some vegetables.

I want a baked potato.

I want a piece of pie.

I want a piece of cake.

I want a dish of ice cream.

I want a cup of coffee.

ORAL READING

Directions: Read these common road signs aloud.

Stop	**Go**
Exit	**Entrance**
No parking	**Curve**
Slow	**Slippery**
Merge	**Yield**
No stopping	**No horns**
Parking meter	**R. R.**
Speed limit	**Right turn on red**
One-way	**No turns**
Fire zone	**Radar zone**
School zone	**Hospital zone**
No U turn	**No entry**
No exit	**Slow down**

ORAL READING

Directions: Read aloud.

I feel sick.

I feel sleepy.

I feel pretty good.

I feel hungry.

I feel tired.

I feel angry.

I feel worried.

I feel upset.

I feel nervous.

I feel happy.

I feel sad.

I feel lonely.

I feel blue.

I feel great.

ORAL READING

Directions: Read aloud.

I have a headache.

I have a pain.

I have a cold.

I have a sore throat.

I have a stomach ache.

I have a sore arm.

I have a sore leg.

I have no money.

I have no patience.

I have a cough.

I have a back ache.

ORAL READING

Directions: Read aloud.

It's a nice day.

It's too cold.

It's cloudy.

It's raining.

It's chilly outside.

It's windy.

It's too hot in here.

It's sunny.

It's cold in this room.

It's too wet to go outside.

It's snowing.

ORAL READING

Directions: Read aloud.

I want to get better.

I want to go home.

I want to go outside.

I want to go to the bathroom.

I want to read the paper.

I want to write a letter.

I want to watch TV.

I want to eat lunch.

I want to see my family.

I want to practice my lesson.

I want to take a walk.

ORAL READING

Directions:　Read aloud.

I need the doctor.

I need a bath.

I need a shave.

I need a blanket.

I need my hair washed.

I need a wash cloth.

I need a tissue.

I need the bedpan.

I need a change of clothes.

I need some money.

I need a rest.

ORAL READING

Directions: Read aloud.

When are you coming back?

When are you leaving?

When will you be ready?

When is he expected?

When are you going?

When will I get better?

When can I go home?

When is he coming over?

When is lunch served?

When is dinner served?

When is breakfast served?

ORAL READING

Directions: Read aloud.

Where are you going?

Where are my shoes?

Where are my friends?

Where is the money?

Where is the nurse?

Where do you live?

Where do you want to go?

Where is the bathroom?

Where is the kitchen?

Where did you go?

Where is my wife/husband?

ORAL READING

Directions: Read aloud.

What time is it?

What do you want?

What am I going to do?

What color is it?

What are you doing?

What time is lunch served?

What time will you be leaving?

What time are you coming?

What is your name?

What is your preference?

What is the matter?

ORAL READING

Directions:　Read aloud.

Who's on the phone?

Who's at the door?

Who's here?

Who's there?

Who's that?

Who's the one?

Who's over there?

Who's ready to go?

Who's next?

Who's he?

Who's that man?

ORAL READING

Directions: Read aloud—household items.

I use a hammer.

I use a broom.

I use a dustpan.

I use a sponge.

I use a mop.

I use a pail.

I use soap.

I use bleach.

I use scissors.

I use a ruler.

I use a scrubbing brush.

ORAL READING

Directions: Read aloud—furniture.

I use a chair.

I use a table.

I use a sofa.

I use a couch.

I use a bed.

I use a blanket.

I use a pillow.

I use a bench.

I use a lamp.

I use a desk.

I use a stool.

I use a shelf.

I use a wheelchair.

ORAL READING

Directions: Read aloud—food items.

I eat bread.

I eat fruit.

I eat eggs.

I eat cake.

I eat steak.

I eat ice cream.

I eat chicken.

I eat fish.

I eat cookies.

I eat potatoes.

I eat vegetables.

I eat toast.

ORAL READING

Directions: Read aloud—useful items.

I use a telephone.

I use a radio.

I use a watch.

I use a toaster.

I use a stove.

I use a needle.

I use thread.

I use a typewriter.

I use a fan.

I use a heater.

I use an air conditioner.

I use a clock-radio.

I use a hanger.

ORAL READING

Directions: Read aloud—ladies' clothing.

I wear a skirt.

I wear a blouse.

I wear a dress.

I wear a top.

I wear slacks.

I wear shoes.

I wear stockings.

I wear a necklace.

I wear earrings.

I wear a bracelet.

I wear a girdle.

I wear a bra.

I wear a slip.

ORAL READING

Directions: Read aloud—men's clothing.

I wear pants.

I wear a shirt.

I wear a tie.

I wear a jacket.

I wear a belt.

I wear a sweater.

I wear shoes.

I wear socks.

I wear shorts.

I wear a T-shirt.

I wear an undershirt.

I wear a suit.

I wear glasses.

ORAL READING

Directions: Read aloud—drinks.

I drink tea.

I drink coffee.

I drink soda.

I drink liquor.

I drink water.

I drink wine.

I drink milk.

I drink beer.

I drink Sanka®.

I drink skim milk.

I drink juice.

I drink iced tea.

I drink diet soda.

BREAKFAST MENU

Directions: Read aloud.

Example: Choose items from each category that you like to eat. Pretend you are speaking to a waitress and use the phrase: "I'LL HAVE SOME ___ ."

orange juice   **bananas**

cantaloupe   **apple cider**

grapefruit juice   **prunes**

Special K®   **Wheatena**®

corn flakes   **oatmeal**

white toast   **rye bread**

rolls   **whole wheat**

scrambled eggs   **poached eggs**

soft-boiled eggs   **ham & eggs**

pancakes   **waffles**

coffee   **tea**   **Sanka**

BREAKFAST MENU

Directions: Read aloud.

Example: Choose items from each category that you like to eat. Pretend you are speaking to a waitress and use the phrase "I'LL HAVE SOME ____."

prune juice   prunes

pineapple juice   grapefruit

melon in season   apricot juice

Rice Krispies®   raisin bran

Ralston®   Farina®

melba toast   crackers

English muffin   pumpernickel

sweet rolls   donuts

cheese omelette   fried eggs

bacon & eggs   **eggs & sausages**

milk   **coffee**   **cocoa**

bouillon   **tea**   **Nescafé®**

LUNCHEON MENU

Directions: Read aloud.

> Example: Choose items from each category that you like to eat. Pretend you are speaking to a waitress and use the phrase "I'LL HAVE SOME _____."

hard-boiled eggs   **vegetable soup**

tuna salad plate   **tomato juice**

bacon, lettuce, & tomato   **egg salad**

ham & cheese   **salmon platter**

Western omelette   **Spanish omelette**

broiled mackerel   **shrimp sandwich**

pie   **cake**

sherbet   **rice pudding**

Coca-Cola®   **milk**

tea   **coffee**

skim milk   **diet sodas**

LUNCHEON MENU

Directions: Read aloud.

Example: Choose items from each category that you like to eat. Pretend you are speaking to a waitress and use the phrase "I'LL HAVE SOME _____."

tossed salad

fruit salad platter

julienne salad

cottage cheese

hamburger

tuna fish sandwich

cheeseburger

grilled cheese

baked fish

egg salad sandwich

mushroom omelette

bacon & eggs

Jell-O

ice cream

custard

Danish pastry

iced tea	iced coffee
diet soda	Sanka
tea	coffee

DINNER MENU

shrimp cocktail	fruit cup
chopped liver	tomato juice
vegetable soup	chicken soup
tossed salad	Caesar salad
Italian dressing	oil & vinegar
filet mignon	lamb chops
roast chicken	meat loaf
pork chops	broiled fish
baked potato	french fries

DINNER MENU

Directions: Read aloud.

Example: Choose items from each category that you like to eat. Pretend you are speaking to a waitress and use the phrase "I'LL HAVE SOME ____."

clam chowder

onion soup

pea soup

mushroom soup

Greek salad

hearts of lettuce

French dressing

house dressing

Roquefort™ dressing

Russian dressing

sirloin steak

sliced turkey

roast beef

lobster

broiled snapper

halibut steak

mashed potatoes

squash

string beans

broccoli

MONEY CONCEPTS

Directions: Read aloud and fill in numerical answers.
Example: A dime equals __10¢__ .

1. A nickel equals _____ .

2. A quarter equals _____ .

3. Four quarters equal _____ .

4. Two dimes and one nickel equal

_____ .

5. Two   ten-dollar   bills   equal

_____ .

6. Five twenty-dollar bills equal

_____ .

7. One   hundred   pennies   equal

_____ .

8. Two nickels equal _____ .

9. Two quarters and dime equal

_____ .

10. Five dimes equal _____ .

11. Three quarters equal _____ .

12. A penny and a quarter equal
    _____.

13. Two dimes and two quarters
    equal _____.

14. Ten dollars and one quarter
    equal _____.

15. Two twenties and three quarters
    equal _____.

MONEY CONCEPTS

Directions: Read written sentences aloud then write corresponding numbers in dollars and cents.

Example: Ten dollars and twenty cents
$10.20

1. One hundred fifty dollars
_____.

2. One thousand five hundred dollars _____.

3. One dollar and fifty-five cents
_____.

4. Twenty dollars and thirty-five cents _____.

5. Three hundred dollars and seventy-five cents _____.

6. Four hundred dollars and ninety-eight cents _____.

7. Nineteen hundred eighty dollars _____.

8. Three thousand five hundred dollars _____.

9. Twelve hundred fifty dollars _____.

10. Eighty-five dollars and ninety-nine cents _____.

11. Forty-four dollars and twenty-five cents _____.
12. Five hundred eighty dollars _____.
13. Fifteen dollars and forty-five cents _____.
14. Seventy-two dollars and fifty cents _____.
15. Nineteen dollars and seventy-nine cents _____.

MONEY CONCEPTS

Directions: Read numbers (dollars and cents) aloud. Then write the amount in longhand.

Example: $150.00 = <u>One hundred fifty dollars</u>

1. $ 10.00 = _____

2. $ 30.00 = _____

3. $ 50.00 = _____ .

4. $ 25.00 = _____

5. $ 75.00 = _____

6. $ 83.00 = _____

7. $115.00 = _____

8. $ 40.50 = _____

9. $ 65.20 = _____

10. $135.10 = _____

11. $210.75 = _____

12. $450.40 = _____

13. $680.62 = _____

14. $349.17 = _____

15. $708.98 = _____

MONEY CONCEPTS

Directions: Read aloud and write the correct answers.

$ .50	$ .65	$ .78	$ .84
+.25	+.22	+.11	+.15

$ 95.00	$ 79.00	$175.00	$356.00
+ 85.00	+ 14.00	+ 98.00	+ 37.00

$ 75.17	$ 35.50	$130.50	$ 10.60
+ 33.52	+ 82.75	+ 95.20	+ 65.60

$ 79.00	$ 85.00	$ 99.00	$ 68.00
− 7.00	− 14.00	− 74.00	− 12.00

$117.00	$159.00	$357.00	$576.00
− 96.63	− 86.48	− 28.96	−123.25

$ 85.75	$ 98.99	$250.25	$315.20
− 25.70	− 35.20	−110.75	− 48.50

TELLING TIME

Directions: Read these times aloud.

Example: <u>1:00 is one o'clock</u>

5:00 = _____ o'clock

4:00 = _____ o'clock

6:00 = _____ o'clock

9:00 = _____ o'clock

1:00 = _____ o'clock

3:00 = _____ o'clock

8:00 = _____ o'clock

10:00 = _____ o'clock

11:00 = _____ o'clock

12:00 = _____ o'clock

7:00 = _____ o'clock

2:00 = _____ o'clock

Use the illustrated clocks on the following page for further practice.

Practice Telling Time

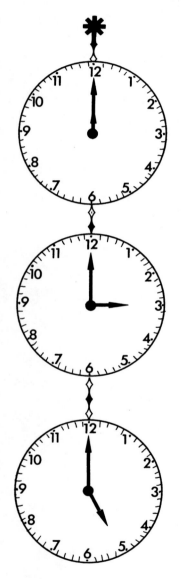

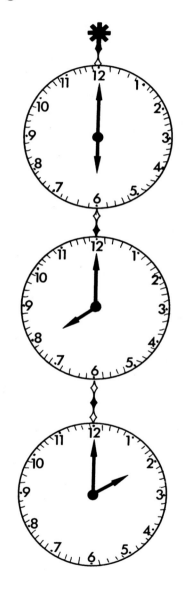

TELLING TIME

Directions: Read these times aloud and then say them in another way.

Example: 4:30 is half-past four

1:30 = half-past _____

12:30 = half-past _____

2:30 = half-past _____

5:30 = half-past _____

6:30 = half-past _____

8:30 = half-past _____

9:30 = half-past _____

4:30 = half-past _____

10:30 = half-past _____

7:30 = half-past _____

3:30 = half-past _____

11:30 = half-past _____

Use the illustrated clocks on the following page for further practice.

Practice Telling Time

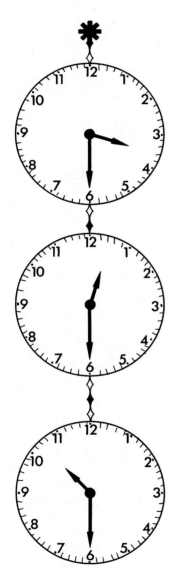

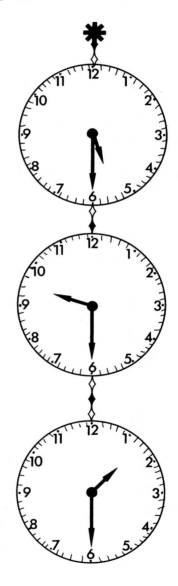

TELLING TIME

Directions: Say these times aloud—o'clock and thirty.

5:00	**4:30**
6:30	**9:00**
7:00	**10:30**
8:30	**11:30**
2:00	**12:00**
1:30	**3:00**
10:00	**7:30**
12:30	**4:00**
11:00	**2:30**
6:00	**5:30**

Use the illustrated clocks on the following page for further practice.

Practice Telling Time

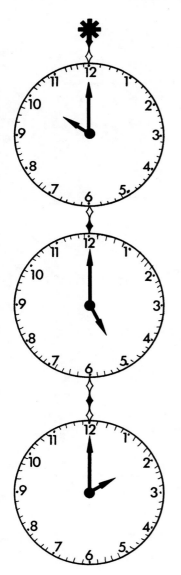

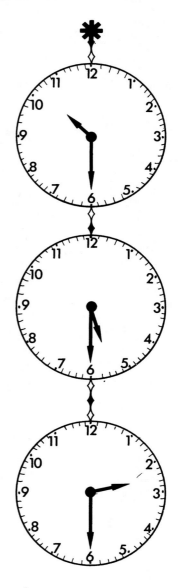

TELLING TIME

Directions: Read these times aloud and then say them in another way.

Example: 5:45 is a quarter of six.

5:45 = a quarter of _____

7:45 = a quarter of _____

8:45 = a quarter of _____

12:45 = a quarter of _____

11:45 = a quarter of _____

10:45 = a quarter of _____

9:45 = a quarter of _____

2:45 = a quarter of _____

4:45 = a quarter of _____

1:45 = a quarter of _____

6:45 = a quarter of _____

3:45 = a quarter of _____

Use the illustrated clocks on the following page for further practice.

Practice Telling Time

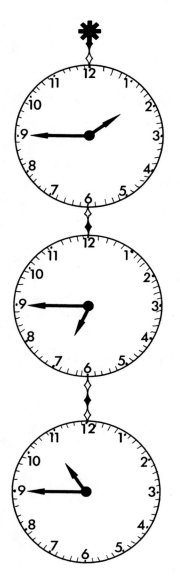
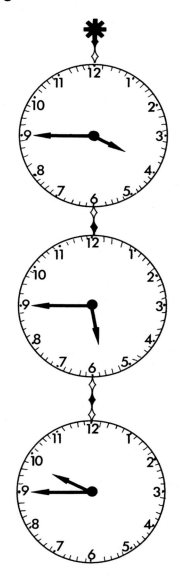

TELLING TIME

Directions: Read these times aloud and then say them in another way.

Example: 5:15 is a quarter after five.

5:15 = a quarter after _____

3:15 = a quarter after _____

1:15 = a quarter after _____

6:15 = a quarter after _____

8:15 = a quarter after _____

10:15 = a quarter after _____

11:15 = a quarter after _____

9:15 = a quarter after _____

7:15 = a quarter after _____

4:15 = a quarter after _____

12:15 = a quarter after _____

Use the illustrated clocks on the following page for further practice.

Practice Telling Time

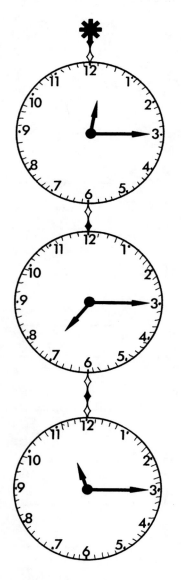
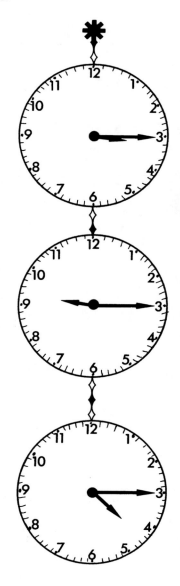

TELLING TIME

Directions: Say these times aloud—15 minutes and 45 minutes.

5:15	**7:45**
6:15	**8:15**
8:45	**2:45**
3:45	**3:15**
1:15	**2:15**
7:15	**6:45**
9:15	**10:45**
12:15	**1:45**
2:45	**4:45**
3:15	**11:45**

Use the illustrated clocks on the following page for further practice.

Practice Telling Time

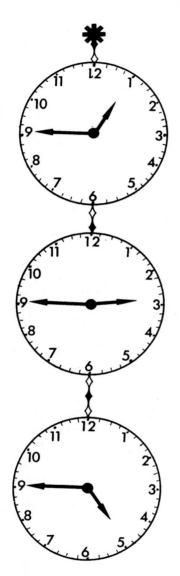
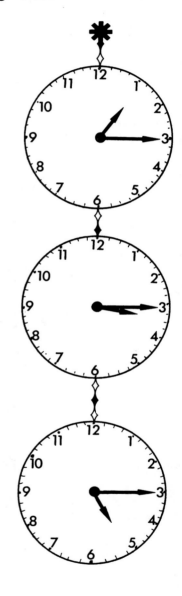

ADVANCED ORAL READING SELECTION

Directions: Read this paragraph, then answer the questions.

Exercising to stay fit is fine but some people are overdoing it. Doctors warn that strenuous exercise, especially in those over forty, may lead to serious and even fatal consequences. Among the exercises of jogging, cycling, swimming and racket sports, swimming was found to be the safest. Some people have died from heart attacks during or shortly after jogging. Many runners complain of aches and pains or some injury to feet, knees and back. Moderate exercise can prolong life and reduce the risk of heart attack for the average person.

1. According to the article, what is the safest exercise for those over forty?
2. What complications may occur from jogging?
3. What should one do to prolong good health?

ADVANCED ORAL READING SELECTION

Directions: Read this paragraph, then answer the questions.

Clipping coupons takes time but it helps save money. Some say you can save from 8% — 20% on a weekly grocery bill. Practically every brand name company offers coupons, but paper items and pet foods have the most offers. The coupons can be found in newspapers, magazines, or on packages. The newspaper's food section carry the largest coupon offerings. In order to maximize savings people have joined clubs to swap coupons — giving away those coupons on items they don't need and exchanging them for desirable ones.

1. Why do people clip food coupons?
2. Where is the best place to find coupon offers?
3. How do people maximize their coupon savings?

ADVANCED ORAL READING SELECTION

Directions: Read this paragraph, then answer the questions.

People like good listeners. To find one is rare. We remember someone who lets us talk our heart out and shows us genuine concern. A bad listener is one who just hears what he wants to hear and doesn't try to understand your feelings. He is impatient, and often doesn't look you in the eye while you're talking. To help comfort someone, encourage them to vent their feelings and think the problem out loud. Then help them focus on what to do next. People aren't born with an ability to listen but one can develop this important skill.

1. What are the qualities of a good listener?
2. What makes a bad listener?
3. How can you help comfort someone who is troubled?

ADVANCED ORAL READING SELECTION

Directions: Read this paragraph, then answer the questions.

Many deaths could be avoided if people knew the basic rules of fire safety. If you live or work in a high-rise building, you should use the fire stairs, not the elevator, in case of fire. When you enter a public place such as a restaurant or hotel, make a habit of noticing the fire exits. Obstructed doorways, lack of sprinklers and overcrowded rooms are common dangers which may lead to disaster. If you smell smoke, sound the alarm and leave the area promptly.

1. **What should you do in a public place to increase your safety?**
2. **Name common fire dangers to be aware of.**
3. **What should you do if you smell smoke?**

ADVANCED ORAL READING SELECTION

Directions: Read this paragraph, then answer the questions.

Why do humans have pets? Some people are lonely. They feel they need something to keep them company. Many people become extremely attached to their animals. Pets provide protection, love and companionship. Some people groom their pets and take great pride in showing them. Other people feel that a pet is too much responsibility. They worry about feeding it, taking care of it while away on vacation and the possibility of it ruining the carpet.

1. What things does a pet provide?
2. Give three disadvantages of owning a pet.
3. Do you own a pet? If so, what kind?

ADVANCED ORAL READING SELECTION

Directions: Read this paragraph, then answer the questions.

If you want a secret hiding place for your valuables and personal documents get a key and safe deposit box. Today there is such a large demand for these boxes that some banks have limited their box rentals to depositors only. Many people who transferred their investments from the stock market into gold, silver, coins, and stamps need a safe place to store their items. There is a greater demand for large-sized safe deposit boxes, because of their capacity to hold precious metals. The bank may not open your box without a court order or without your approval.

1. What items are usually stored in safe deposit boxes?
2. Why has the demand for larger boxes increased?
3. By what means can the bank open your box without your approval?

ADVANCED ORAL READING SELECTION

Directions: Read this paragraph, then answer the questions.

Choosing the right travel agent is very important. It may help save you precious time and money. A good travel agent can suggest the lowest airfares, best cruise schedules, hotel accommodations and tour itineraries. A good way to choose an agent is through the recommendation of a satisfied friend. Agents may vary widely in competence and honesty. They earn their money primarily from commissions paid by tour wholesalers, hotels and transportation carriers, so that theoretically you pay nothing for their services.

1. What are the chief functions of a travel agent?
2. What is the best way to choose a travel agent?
3. How do agents earn their money?

ADVANCED ORAL READING SELECTION

Directions: Read this paragraph, then answer the questions.

What should labels tell us about prescription drugs? Labels should state the benefits of drug actions and possible risks of the medication. All drugs may have side-effects. Even aspirin can cause gastric bleeding in some people. The way drugs react in the human body may differ depending on a person's age, weight and overall health. Some drugs and foods in combination may cause ill side-effects. One objection to more detailed labeling is increased cost due to printing.

1. **What important information should be included on a label?**
2. **What factors may influence drug reactions?**
3. **What is one drawback of more detailed labeling?**

ADVANCED ORAL READING SELECTION

Directions: Read this paragraph, then answer the questions.

Anyone who is planning to stay as a guest in someone's house for three days or more ought to help his host feel at ease. The most helpful way is to plan frequent absences from the house. These should be announced in advance. If necessary, the guest should invent excuses and go off by himself to give the family opportunities to relax in privacy. If arguments occur the guest should try to ignore them and not take sides. The guest should help clean up. A small gift might also be appropriate.

1. What is the most helpful way to help a host feel at ease?
2. In what ways can a guest show his appreciation?
3. What should one do in case of an argument?

ADVANCED ORAL READING SELECTION

Directions: Read this paragraph, then answer the questions.

Night after night, families spend their prime time watching television. According to a recent poll, the average viewing time of the American child between six and sixteen years of age is 20-24 hours per week. Many parents do not restrict either the type of program or the number of hours watched. Money was the subject husbands and wives argued most about. Television was a strong contender, especially when to turn it off and which programs to watch. The family has less time for sharing and communicating when they watch too much television.

1. What is the average number of hours per week that children watch T.V.?
2. What subject did husbands and wives argue most about?
3. Name some disadvantages of too much T.V. watching.

ADVANCED ORAL READING SELECTION

Directions: Read this paragraph, then answer the questions.

A gift certificate for a bargain vacation may come in the mail or in a newspaper ad. The offer sounds very exciting — a fun-filled vacation for two in Las Vegas or Miami. For a low $15.00 fee you are entitled to two nights lodging and meals worth approximately $350.00 per couple. After paying the $15.00 a Chicago man was advised that his gift certificate would not become valid until he bought his round-trip airfare from a specified travel agency. After sending his check he was told to pick up his tickets at the airport. On arrival, to his dismay, he found the airlines showed no record of his reservations.

1. Where might you find an offer for a bargain vacation?
2. Where was the vacation offered?
3. What happened at the airport?

ADVANCED ORAL READING SELECTION

Directions: Read this story aloud, then answer questions about the paragraph.

Requiring exact fare on buses has accomplished its goal of reducing robberies and violence. There were 948 robberies or acts of violence on buses four years ago and only two this year. Also, drivers estimate that riders without the proper change put in an additional fifteen to fifty cents a day per bus in the fare boxes. This has provided $5,000 extra income since the program began.

1. Has exact fare reduced the crime level?

2. What other advantages has exact fare created for the bus company?

3. What can a passenger do if he doesn't have exact change?

4. What do you think of this new system?

ADVANCED ORAL READING SELECTION

Directions: Read this paragraph, then answer the questions.

"Maybe someday, if I have the time," is something we have all said at one time or another. No one man has more hours in the day than another, however, time must be used wisely. Your "own time" is under your personal control, and your "work time" is controlled by others. The best way to manage your own time is to make a list and assign priorities. Do top priority matters first — keep working on one item until you finish it. While on the job, avoid time-wasting phone conversations and calling meetings that have no purpose.

1. What are the two categories of time?
2. What is the best way to manage your "own time"?
3. How can you avoid wasting time on the job?

ADVANCED ORAL READING SELECTION

Directions: Read this story aloud, then answer questions about the paragraph.

Mrs. Helen Rubin was taking her driving test when she drove her husband's new car into a seven foot deep river. After she and her examiner were rescued, the examiner was asked if she had failed her test. "We don't know yet," he answered, "She didn't finish it."

1. Where did she drive her car?

2. Was she rescued?

3. Did Mrs. Rubin pass her test?

4. Retell this story in your own words.

ADVANCED ORAL READING SELECTION

Directions: Read this paragraph, then answer the questions.

An innkeeper who owns beach-front property adjacent to Plymouth Rock wanted the small rocks that covered his beach removed. Instead of incurring the expense of having them removed, he posted a sign for tourists which read "Take home an honest-to-goodness Plymouth Rock." His beach is clear now, and he is thinking of importing more rocks to keep the tourists happy.

1. What did the innkeeper want changed about his beachfront property?

2. How did he accomplish this change without paying for it?

3. How is he planning to keep the tourists happy?

4. Retell in your own words.

ADVANCED ORAL READING SELECTION

Directions: Read this story aloud, then answer questions about the paragraph.

A train passenger was asked why he pulled the emergency cord to stop the train. He said that he had spotted a beautiful blonde at the station. He got on the train himself because he thought he saw her boarding. When he discovered that she wasn't on board, he pulled the cord that halted the train so that he could walk back to the station to look for her.

1. Who halted the train?

2. Why?

3. What did he do after the train stopped?

4. Retell in your own words.

ADVANCED ORAL READING SELECTION

Directions: Read this story aloud, then answer questions about the paragraph.

A salesman, John Brenner, who was passing through Pittsburgh in a car, was struck by a Port Authority maintenance truck. When he went across the street to a service station to report the accident, he walked into a holdup. The robber took about $40 from his wallet and an undetermined amount from the station attendant.

1. What kind of vehicle struck John Brenner's car?

2. Where did he go to report the accident?

3. What happened to him while he was in the service station?

4. Retell this story in your own words.

ADVANCED ORAL READING SELECTION

Directions: Read this paragraph, then answer these questions.

The Wilsons will be suspicious the next time a man says there is a telegram for them. They were robbed at their home by a man who was supposedly delivering a telegram. As Mr. Wilson called his wife to the door to sign for the message, the robber drew his gun and demanded money. Then he struck Mr. Wilson and threw him to the floor. Mrs. Wilson's screams attracted a neighbor across the street, who phoned the police. The gunman's two partners were waiting in a car across the street. They yelled to the robber to hurry and retreat. Only Mrs. Wilson's wedding ring was taken before he ran off. The police arrived and the trio was arrested after they were spotted heading west on 109th street in a 1969 red 2-door Chevrolet.

1. What excuse did the robber give to gain entry into the house?

2. What happened when Mrs. Wilson screamed?

3. What valuables did the robber take?

4. How many men were involved?

5. What kind of car was the getaway car?

6. Retell the story in your own words.

WRITING DEVELOPMENT SKILLS

A) Copying

B) Writing to dictation

C) Writing from memory

D) Advanced writing

WRITING DEVELOPMENT
SKILLS

THERE IS SOME CONTROVERSY as to whether or not a speech
pathologist should include practicing writing skills in the
therapeutic management of the aphasic patient. In regard to
this question, it has often been the responsibility of the occu-
pational or physical therapist to teach writing because of the
muscular weakness in the patient's hand. Writing therapy
under these conditions is directed toward improving motor
control.

However, although there may be muscular weakness in the
hand of the stoke victim, more often the patient's writing
difficulties are due to a breakdown in the word-recall process.
This symbolic dysfunction may be manifested by substitution,
perseveration, omission, and reversals of letters. Consequently, practicing writing skills logically falls within the
domain of the speech pathologist.

Practicing writing skills can be beneficial to the patient in
the following ways: First of all, some patients cannot make
themselves understood adequately because of reduced vocabulary. However, these patients may be able to provide enough
clues through writing to enable the listener to comprehend
some of their communication attempts. Therefore, writing
provides the patient with an alternate means of communication. For example, the patient may write "Calll the doctr."
Although there are obvious agraphic errors, the message is still
discernible.

Second, having patients trace and copy words as well as

writing from memory and dictation can be helpful in expanding vocabulary recall.

Third, it is most useful for the patient to learn how to sign his own name. Oftentimes his signature will be needed on important papers.

Finally, being able to accurately copy words and being able to write one's own name gives the patient a psychological boost. Such a lift is important in counteracting the frustration and depression that most patients feel in trying to regain communications skills.

The procedure for practicing writing skills is as follows: First, the patient's ability to hold the pencil must be evaluated. Very often one arm or hand is weakend or paralyzed as a result of the brain injury. If the patient is unable to grasp the pencil in his affected hand, he must be shown how to write using the unaffected hand. Proper pencil grip, positioning of paper, and hand placement on table must be shown to the aphasic patient. The patient should be seated upright in a chair and should rest his arm, including the elbow, on the table. A clipboard should be used, The heel of the hand gripping the pencil should be resting on the table too. Often patients make the mistake of holding the pencil at the end with the hand suspended in midair. There is no hand stability and therefore handwriting legibility is poor.

Second, with the hand in the proper position, the patient is given a pencil and asked to write his name from memory. If he is unable to do this, begin with copying exercises. Have him copy a straight line, then a circle, then the numbers 1—2—3. Next, print his name in capitals and have him copy it. If he has difficuty, have him trace each letter individually and copy the individual letters behind the original. If he is unable to do this, the clinician should draw the letters of his name with broken lines and instruct the patient to connect the lines to form the letters. When he is able to copy printed letters, the patient is asked to copy script. A felt-tip pen available in most stationery stores, is often helpful since the ink flows evenly and it does not require any significant amount of pressure. After the patient is able to write with the felt-tip pen, a regular ball-point pen is introduced.

Further practice in copying or words, phrases, and sentences should be accomplished before proceeding to writing from dictation.

Ask patient to write simple words to dictation. Say a word, then use the word in a sentence, e.g. say "Write the word DOOR—Open the front DOOR." If the patient is unable to write the word from dictation, have him copy it first.

After the patient is able to write from dictation, have the patient practice writing words from memory. Show the patient a picture of a useful item such as "COMB," or use the real object, i.e. hold up a comb—have him write the word corresponding to the item presented, then have him write the word corresponding to the item presented, then have him read the word aloud. Use the illustrations of Useful Objects in Categories in Section Three pages 182 to 207 for the practice. Have the patient practice writing a word from memory that corresponds to the picture you show to him. Then, have him practice writing an appropriate word to complete the thought of the fill-in sentences in this section and those in Section Three. Next the patient is given a single word and told to write a sentence using the key word.

When the patient has reached this level of achievement, the final tasks are reading paragraphs aloud and writing paraphrases of the contents of the paragraphs. Any exercise in which the patient must generate sentences on his own are appropriate, e.g. writing letters, shopping lists, and reminder notes, etc.

Thus, practicing writing can also aid in the recall of verbal language.

COPYING

Directions: Have patient practice tracing these forms, then try
to copy them.

A Circle   **A Straight Line**

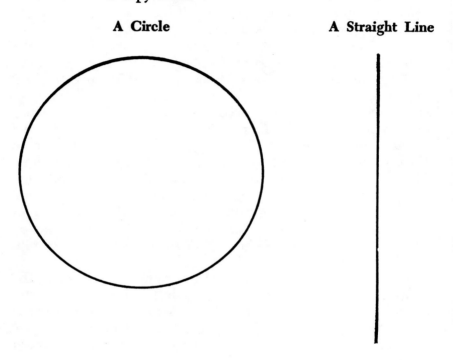

COPY THE NUMBERS

1	2	3
4	5	6
7	8	9
10	11	12

COPY THE NUMBERS

1	30	17
25	4	55
6	83	9
100	52	275

COPY YOUR NAME

Directions: Trace each letter in your name—one at a time; then, copy it below. (Clinician should print the patient's name below in large capitals). When the patient can print, have him practice script writing.

COPY YOUR NAME

Directions: If a patient cannot copy letters in his name by tracing and copying below, the clinician should draw the letters with broken lines and have patient connect the broken lines to form the letter.

Example: If the name to be copied is JACK draw the letters with broken lines as below:

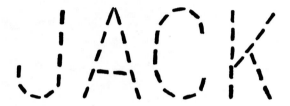

Repeat this procedure several times for both his first and last name.

When the patient can connect the lines to form the complete letters, have him copy the letters below without assistance.

COPY THESE WORDS

door

comb

house

key

tissue

cup

COPY

Directions: Copy these sentences on a separate piece of paper:

Open the door.

Comb your hair.

Come over to my house.

Give me the key.

I need a tissue.

I want a cup of coffee.

Turn on the light, please.

Close the window over there.

Who's on the telephone?

I need my glasses.

WRITE TO DICTATION

Directions: The clinician recites the numbers as patient writes
them down:

1.   5   3   4

2.   6   7   2

3.   9   4   9   1

4.   8   7   1   1

5.   6   7   4   2   2

6.   6   7   3   0   1

7.   7   5   7   1   8   4

8.   5   3   4   3   6   7   6

9.   8   8   7   7   3   8   1

10.   8   5   4   3   5   4   5

WRITE TO DICTATION

Directions: The clinician says each word aloud—as the patient writes to dictation.

cup

key

comb

bed

chair

table

phone

WRITE TO DICTATION

Directions: Say these phrases aloud—as patient writes them down.

1. to the house

2. at the door

3. on the phone

4. to the doctor

5. in the car

6. to the bathroom

7. to the store

8. with a key

9. with a knife

10. in the cup

WRITE FROM DICTATION

Directions: The clinician says the numbers below and the patient writes them from dictation.

phone numbers:

893–0924	**534–3676**
574–1039	**866–6671**
873–1121	**853–9949**
674–1021	**325–0461**

addresses:

25 West 34 St.	**3311 Long St.**
995 East 7 St.	**7741 Brown Ave.**
11 N.E. 191 St.	**141–08 Rock Blvd.**
320 S.W. 88 Ave.	**9250 Maple Rd.**

WRITING FROM MEMORY

Directions: Have the patient write his own name, address, and phone number from memory.

Practice writing your:

name

address

phone number

names of family members

WRITING WORDS FROM MEMORY

Use the illustrations of useful items in categories in Section Three, pages 182 to 207. Have the patient look at each picture— say the name of the picture aloud and then have him try to write the name of the illustration from memory. If he is unable to do this have him write the word as you spell the letters individually, to him. If the patient is still unsuccessful, write the word for him and have him copy it several times. After copying it, have him try to write the word from memory.

WRITING FROM MEMORY

FINISH THESE SENTENCES

Directions: Write in any appropriate word to complete the thought.

Example: **I am ___tired___ .**

I need _____.

I like _____.

I was _____.

I drink _____.

I eat _____.

I watch _____.

I went _____.

I use _____.

I have _____.

I take _____.

I call _____.

I go _____.

I want _____.

SPONTANEOUS WRITING

Directions: Write a sentence using these words:

1. **knife**

2. **coffee**

3. **bread**

4. **door**

5. **phone**

6. **bathroom**

7. **doctor**

8. **store**

9. **newspaper**

10. **car**

SPONTANEOUS WRITING

Directions: Write a sentence using these words:

1. **read**

2. **talk**

3. **drink**

4. **go**

5. **open**

6. **take**

7. **eat**

8. **sleep**

9. **write**

10. **want**

SPONTANEOUS WRITING

Directions: Write a sentence for each verb:

Example: **cut**   <u>I cut my finger.</u>

blow   _____

sit   _____

watch   _____

fell down   _____

cry   _____

fish   _____

wait   _____

play   _____

cash   _____

catch   _____

wash   _____

SPONTANEOUS WRITING

Directions: Write a sentence using each verb:

Example: **drink**   I drink coffee.
_____

eat   _____

hold   _____

buy   _____

make   _____

fry   _____

boil   _____

serve   _____

come   _____

sign   _____

leave   _____

shop   _____

SPONTANEOUS WRITING

Directions: Have the patient practice the following items:

1. **Practice writing a letter to a close relative or friend.**

2. **Practice writing a shopping list.**

3. **Practice writing down names and telephone numbers of close friends—as many as you can remember (refer to your personal phone book).**

4. **Practice writing a thank-you note.**

5. **Practice writing daily reminders of appointments.**

CONCLUSION

Most authorities in the field of speech pathology agree that, in addition to the spontaneous recovery that occurs following an injury to the brain, a carefully structured treatment program consisting of repetition and practice exercises can greatly enhance the possibility of recovery of functional speech and language skills. Recovery includes improvement in comprehension, reading, writing, and speech and language skills. Just how much recovery can take place varies with each case and usually depends upon the scope and the severity of the initial injury, the patient's motivational level, and the support of family members and the speech pathologist.

The questions that are asked most often are (1) How long will the recovery take? and (2) How much improvement can be expected? These are difficult questions to answer.

TIME NEEDED FOR RECOVERY

The length of time for maximum recovery varies, depending mostly on the severity of the brain injury. Some patients with minimal brain damage, e.g. mild slurring of speech, recover fully in a few weeks. Some patients with massive brain damage, e.g. those who are unable to comprehend any simple commands, usually make some improvement but it is slow and gradual over the course of approximately a year or more. Based on personal experience, most patients do show improvement in the recovery of language skills in about three to six months following the brain injury, up to approximately one and a half years; i.e. many patients progress from being able to repeat sounds, to saying simple words, to using simple sentences within that time. Some patients continue to make observable progress even after a year or two poststroke. In those cases, aphasia rehabilitation should be continued.

LIMITS OF IMPROVEMENT

It is generally agreed that most patients improve to some degree; even the most severely impaired, i.e. those with irretrievable oral musculature impairment or profound comprehension impairment, may be able to learn to communicate in a nonverbal way through gestures or by using a communication board. Others may progress to a full return of language skills with no noticeable residual deficit at all. The majority learn to communicate basic needs and to carry on a simple conversation. Some unfortunately remain essentially noncommunicative.

I have been surprised myself sometimes by the success of patients who initially appear very severely involved when first seen in the hospital a short time after the onset of brain injury. Until the patient is neurologically stable, which will be determined by the physician, no definite prognosis can be made. If a patient can understand simple commands and matching tasks, one can be more optimistic regarding recovery of basic communication skills with speech pathology treatment.

It is the purpose of this manual to help guide the speech pathologist and untrained family members who want to help the aphasic patient by providing structured practice material to facilitate the relearning of language. The author encourages the clinician to use his ingenuity to improvise and adapt these materials to fit the patient's particular interests and needs.

SUGGESTED REFERENCES AND FURTHER READINGS

1. Agranowitz, Aleen and McKeown, Milfred R.: *Aphasia Handbook.* Springfield, Thomas, 1964.
2. American Heart Assoc. (Publication DM 359) *Aphasia and the Family.* Single copies available free from your local heart association.
3. American Heart Assoc. (Publication EM 294) *Strokes: A Guide for the Family.* Single copies available free from your local heart association.
4. Benson, Frank and Geschwind, Norman: Aphasias and related disturbances. In Baker, A. B. (Ed.). *Clinical Neurology,* 3rd ed. New York, Hoeber, 1971, Vol. 1, Chap. 8.
5. Boone, Daniel R.: *An Adult Has Aphasia* (pamphlet). Danville, Ill., Interstate Printers & Publishers, Inc., 1965.
6. Buck, McKenzie: *Dysphasia: Professional Guidance for Family and Patient,* Englewood Cliffs, New Jersey, Prentice-Hall, 1968.
7. Cooper, Morton: *Modern Techniques of Vocal Rehabilitation,* Springfield, Thomas, 1973.
8. Dolch, E. W.: *Basic Sight Vocabulary Cards,* Champaign, Ill., Garrard, 1949.
9. Eisenson, Jon: *Adult Aphasia,* New York, Appleton, 1973.
10. Eisenson, Jon: Aphasia in adults, In Travis, L. E. (Ed.). *Handbook of Speech Pathology and Audiology,* New York, Appleton, 1971, Chap. 48-50.
11. Eisenson, Jon: *Examining for Aphasia.* New York, Psychological Corp., 1954.
12. Gardner, Warren: *Left-handed Writing, Instruction Manual,* Danville, Ill., Interstate Printers & Publishers, Inc. 1958.
13. Geschwind, N.: Varieties of naming errors. *Cortex, 3:*97-112, 1967.
14. Goodglass, H. and Hunt, J.: Grammatical complexity and aphasic speech. *Word, 14:*197-207, 1958.
15. Goodglass, H. and Mayer, J.: Agrammatism in Aphasia. *Speech Hearing Disorders, 23:*99-111, 1958.
16. Head, H.: *Aphasia and Kindred Disorders of Speech,* New York, Macmillan, 1926.
17. Longerrich, Mary C.: *Manual for the Aphasia Patient,* New York, Macmillan, 1958.
18. Nielsen, J. M.: *Agnosia, Apraxia, Aphasia: Their Value in Cerebral Localization,* 2nd ed. New York, Hoerber, 1946.
19. Osgood, C. E. and Miron, M. S. (Eds.), *Approaches to the Study of Aphasia.* Urbana, Univ. Illinois Press, 1963.
20. Penfield, W. and Roberts, L.: *Speech and Brain-Mechanisms.* Princeton, N.J., Princeton University Press. 1959.
21. Porch, Bruce: *Porch Index of Communicative Abilities,* Palo Alto, California, Consulting Psychologist Press, 1967, Vol. 2.

22. Sarno, John E. and Sarno, Martha Taylor: *Stroke—the Condition and the Patient.* New York, McGraw-Hill, 1969.
23. Schuell, Hildred, Jenkins, James, and Jiménez-Pabón, Edward: *Aphasia in Adults: Diagnosis, Prognosis and Therapy,* 2nd ed. New York, Harper & Row, 1965.
24. Schuell, H.: *Aphasia Theory and Therapy.* Baltimore, University Park Press, 1974.
25. Schuell, H., Jenkins, J. J., and Carroll, J. B.: A factor analysis of the Minnesota test for diff, diag. of aphasia. *J. Speech Hear. Res.,* 5:349-369.
26. Sheehan, Vivian: Rehabilitation of aphasics in an army hospital. *J. Speech Disorders, 11:*149-157, 1946.
27. Sies, L. F.: Aphasia and general semantics. *ETC, 26:*116-118, 1964.
28. Sies, L. F. and Butler, R. F.: A personal account of dysphasia. *J Speech Hear. Disorders, 28:*261-266, 1964.
29. Speech & Language Materials, Inc., P.O. Box 721, Tulsa, Oklahoma, 74101. Useful items, Photo Sequence Cards, etc.
30. Taylor, Martha L.: *Understanding Aphasia: A Guide for Family and Friends* (pamphlet). Available from Institute of Rehabilitation Medicine, New York University Medical Center, 400 East 34 St., New York, N.Y., 10016, 1958.
31. Taylor, Martha L. and Marks, Morton M.: *Aphasia Rehabilitation Manual and Therapy Kit,* New York, McGraw-Hill, 1959.
32. Wepman, Joseph: *Recovery from Aphasia.* New York, Ronald Press, 1951.
33. Word Making Productions, P.O. Box 305, Salt Lake City, Utah.

INDEX

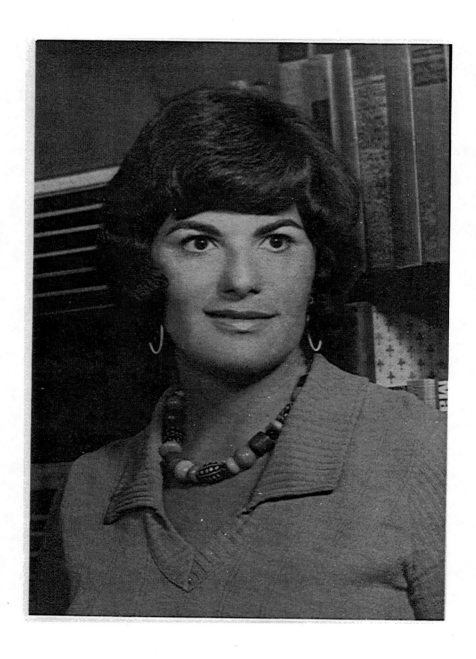

ABOUT THE AUTHOR . . .

Stephanie Stryker received her bachelor's degree in Education from the University of Miami, Florida, and her M.A. in Speech Pathology and Audiology from New York University. Her professional experience includes service as itinerant speech clinician with the Dade County Public Schools and as instructor for adult aphasics and cleft palate patients in the Department of Audiology-Speech Pathology of the University of Miami School of Medicine. Ms. Stryker is currently in private practice in Miami Beach, Florida. She concentrates on the treatment of adult brain-injury, laryngectomy and voice patients. She also acts as consultant to seven major hospitals in the Miami area and is affiliated with several nursing home and home health agencies. She is a licensed speech pathologist in the state of Florida and holds a Certificate of Clinical Competence in Speech Pathology.